ABOUT THE BOOK

Discover a five-point plan for overcoming anxiety, depression, and addiction. Learn the symptoms, causes, treatment, and relapse prevention strategies that will improve your life. You will learn how stress management and cognitive therapy can help you and step-by-step instructions on how to use them.

Discover how your thinking affects your quality of life. You will learn why dwelling on the few negatives in your life and ignoring the positives makes you prone to anxiety, depression, and addiction. Also learn how thinking that things have to be perfect, and being hard on yourself, can lead to trouble. Learn strategies for overcoming these negative habits and how not to repeat them in the future.

Dr. Melemis is a leading expert in addiction and mood disorders. He learned the importance of stress management and cognitive therapy after being diagnosed with cancer while in medical school. During the past twenty years, he has taught these techniques and seen how they improve people's lives. The book contains numerous exercises and a one-month step-by-step program to get you started. If you follow the simple steps in this book, you will be on your way to transforming your life.

PRAISE FOR
I WANT TO CHANGE MY LIFE

Winner of the Gordon Bell Award for Journalism in 2010

"This book is so clearly and beautifully crafted that just reading it reduces tension. Dr. Melemis has taken a complex subject and distilled it into pure therapeutic magic. Put simply: this book will heal you."
– **Hugh Prather**, author of *Notes to Myself*

"When treating the problems of life, put this book in the first-aid kit."
– **A. James Giannini**, MD, FCP, DFAPA, FRSM
Director, Substance Abuse Services, CMHC of Middle Georgia
Formerly: Director, ASC, Yale University
Formerly: Professor, Psychiatry, Ohio State University

"This book could prove very beneficial to many people. I especially like the distinction between stress and tension and the clear instructions on how to engage in the various practices of relaxation."
– **Thupten Jinpa**, official translator to the **Dalai Lama**

I WANT TO CHANGE MY LIFE

I WANT TO CHANGE MY LIFE

HOW TO OVERCOME ANXIETY, DEPRESSION & ADDICTION

STEVEN M. MELEMIS PhD MD

Modern Therapies
Toronto

Contact Modern Therapies through www.moderntherapies.com
Modern Therapies is a registered trademark of Modern Therapies Ltd.

Library and Archives Canada Cataloguing in Publication

Melemis, Steven M. (Steven Michael), 1952-
I want to change my life : how to overcome anxiety, depression, and addiction / Steven M. Melemis.

Includes bibliographical references and index.
ISBN 978-1-897572-23-8
1. Self-actualization (Psychology).
2. Anxiety disorders--Popular works.
3. Depression, Mental--Popular works.
4. Substance abuse--Popular works.
5. Stress management--Popular works. I. Title.

BF637.S4M46 2010   158.1   C2009-907390-0

Book Design: Jennifer Stimson Design
Author's photo: Edward Gajdel
Printed in the United States

CONTENTS

INTRODUCTION

The purpose of life is the pursuit of happiness. But sometimes you can lose your way and find yourself on the wrong path. When that happens, how do you change the course of your life? This book will show you how to improve your life, and give you the coping skills to achieve your goals.

The focus of this book is on how to overcome anxiety, depression, and addiction. They are the most common mental health problems we face, and they share similar causes and similar treatments. They are also interconnected. If you have one of these conditions, you are more likely to have another. This is especially true for addiction, where people who suffer from anxiety or depression are sometimes driven to addiction as a form of self-medication.

The book is based on a five-point plan for change. You will discover what you need to change, learn new coping skills, and see how to incorporate these skills into your life. You will also learn how to avoid repeating old habits so that the changes you make will stick.

The two most important things people need to change in order to improve their lives are stress and negative thinking. Common examples of stress are dwelling on fears, resentments, and on the past. Most stress comes from within.

The most common type of negative thinking is all-or-nothing thinking. Do you think that things have to be perfect, and anything less is a failure? Do you focus on the few negatives in your life and ignore the many positives? You will learn why this puts you at higher risk for anxiety, depression, and addiction.

I have specialized in addiction medicine and mood disorders for over 20 years, and I have seen how stress and negative thinking destroy people's lives. Many of my patients are doctors, lawyers, and nurses who are referred to me because they have run into trouble. I also treat a broad range of patients at a drug rehab hospital. It's clear that people's problems are the same no matter what their job or how much money they make.

The consequences of stress and negative thinking are everywhere. Anxiety and depression are on the rise. Addiction is a growing epidemic. Relationships are suffering. People's health is suffering. This is a wakeup call to the nature of these problems and a strategy for overcoming them. If you follow the simple steps in this book, I am confident that within a month you will begin to improve your life.

The Story Behind the Book

I'd like to tell you how this book got started. Two months after beginning medical school, I was diagnosed with cancer. I was treated with surgery followed by months of radiation. Then the doctors told me that if I could survive the next five years I would be considered cured. I don't think I was consciously worried about dying, but the stress of my diagnosis plus medical school eventually gave me an ulcer. I needed to learn to relax.

I bought a few books on meditation, hoping they would help. But I found them either vague or mystical. I was heading into my medical exams with what felt like a hot coal in my stomach. I needed practical advice.

Eventually I pieced together the common elements in all the meditation books I had read, and began practicing this technique. Once I adopted that simple approach, I was amazed at how quickly I started to feel better.

Surviving cancer was both terrifying and liberating. It reminded me that we are on this world for only a short time, and we shouldn't waste it. After graduating from medical school, I began teaching stress management to my patients, since many of the problems they faced were due to stress. At first, I was worried that they might think I was too far out there. But many of them gave it a try, and most of them found it helpful.

I called my approach mind-body relaxation and eventually I began to lecture on it. People would often come up to me and ask me if there were any books on the subject I could recommend. That's when I remembered the advice of Toni Morrison: "If there's a book you really want to read, but it hasn't been written yet, then you must write it." That was the beginning of this book. It has taken ten years to finish it.

How the Book Is Organized

The book is divided into two parts. The first half introduces the basic coping skills of change: mind-body relaxation and cognitive therapy. The second half shows you how to use those coping skills.

I begin with the basic five-point plan for change. You will learn why mind-body relaxation and cognitive therapy are important for change and how they can be used together. You will learn an expanded version of cognitive therapy that allows you to look deeper into your negative thinking and make lasting changes.

In a sense, these represent the Eastern and Western approaches to self-help. They are the best of modern medicine combined with mindful meditation, stress management, psychology and cognitive therapy to produce a simple and effective strategy for transforming your life. The first half of the book ends with a one-month step-by-step program that ties it all together.

In the second half of the book you will learn how to use the coping skills from the first half. Not every chapter will apply to you. This half begins with a section called "Life" that looks at self-esteem, health, and relationships. Everyone can benefit from improving these issues.

But if you picked up this book specifically to overcome anxiety, depression, or addiction, this section will be particularly helpful to you. Anxiety, depression, and addiction impact every aspect of life and leave behind a swath of destruction. Once you have begun to improve your particular problem, you will still have to clean up the impact left behind. These chapters will show you how to repair the rest of your life.

The next three chapters deal with the broad topic of anxiety, including panic attacks and post-traumatic stress disorder. You will learn the symptoms, causes, treatment, and relapse prevention strategies. Each chapter includes exercises to increase your understanding.

The next three chapters focus on depression. You will learn the causes, treatment, and relapse prevention strategies. This section builds on the anxiety chapters because many people who suffer from depression also suffer from anxiety.

The next section looks at addiction. There is a long chapter called "The Five Rules of Recovery," which explains the five most important things you need to do in order to recover. I developed these rules while trying to understand why some people do well in recovery, while others don't. It has become one of my most requested lectures. These chapters build on the techniques you learned in the anxiety and depression chapters.

This book is an optimistic message for anyone who suffers from anxiety, depression, or addiction. You are not alone. You can change your life. Many people have succeeded and are now enjoying better lives. You can do it too.

For more information on these issues, you can refer to the supplementary websites that I have written to complement this book:
www.AnxietyDepressionHealth.org
www.AddictionsAndRecovery.org
www.CognitiveTherapyGuide.org
www.StressRelaxationGuide.org.

May this book bring you peace, happiness, and good health.

1

A FIVE-POINT PLAN
FOR CHANGE

"I believe that the very purpose of our life is to seek happiness.... One begins by identifying those factors which lead to happiness and those which lead to suffering. Having done this, one then sets about gradually eliminating those factors which lead to suffering and cultivating those which lead to happiness." [1] – THE DALAI LAMA

Happiness is an inside job. To improve the quality of your life, you must start by looking at yourself. No doubt, external factors play a role in overall happiness. But most external factors cannot be changed, and those that can rarely play a major role. If you don't change who you are, any changes you make will feel nice temporarily, but then you'll go back to feeling the way you did before.

In this chapter, you will learn the five basic points of change that are used throughout the book. You will learn how to improve your life from the inside out.

1. Get ready for change
2. Identify what you need to change
3. Let go of old habits to make room for change
4. Learn new coping skills
5. Incorporate the changes into your life

Get Ready for Change

Don't be afraid to look at yourself. It is almost certain you will find a few things that you don't like. Everyone has a few dark corners in their character. That's normal. It's not scary, and shouldn't be an obstacle to change.

Looking at yourself is liberating. There are only a few things you need to change in order to make big improvements in your life. Start with your easiest issues, and you will gradually make changes in the rest because everything in your life is connected.

Take small steps. Don't take an all-or-nothing approach to change and sabotage yourself before you start. Don't try to change your life all at once. An all-or-nothing approach is overwhelming because it's hard to make big changes, and you don't see the significance of small changes, so you end up doing nothing. Decide ahead of time to take small steps, and you will make progress. The techniques in this book are designed to work at whatever pace you choose.

Identify What You Need to Change

Stress and negative thinking are the most important things you need to change. Examples of stress include fears, resentments, dwelling on the past, or worrying about the future. Examples of negative thinking include all-or-nothing thinking and disqualifying the positives.

Do you think that things have to be perfect, and anything less is a failure? Do you focus on the few negatives in your life and ignore the many positives? This kind of thinking leads to most cases of unhappiness, and in more serious cases leads to anxiety, depression, and addiction.

How does all-or-nothing thinking lead to problems? If you think that everything you do has to be perfect, you are bound to feel anxious because you don't allow yourself to make mistakes, which is a normal part of progress. Perhaps you're afraid that if you make a mistake you'll be criticized, or that people won't like you, or you'll seem flawed.

It can lead to depression because if you think you have to be perfect, you feel trapped by your own high standards, which is exhausting. All-or-nothing thinking can lead to addiction because anxiety and depression feel so uncomfortable that you may think of turning to drugs or alcohol to escape. In Chapters 2 and 3, you will learn more about how stress and negative thinking lead to anxiety, depression, and addiction.

Make Room for Change

The most overlooked part of change is making room for change. This is the missing piece in most self-help plans, and the reason why many people fail. They focus on why they are unhappy, thinking that this alone will lead to change. But this is just one part of change. The missing part is letting go of old habits so that you don't repeat the same mistakes. If focusing on why you're unhappy was enough, you'd be happy by now.

When you're tense, you tend to do what's familiar and wrong instead of what's new and right. This explains why you tend to repeat mistakes. When you're tense, your ego, fears, and anxious mind get in the way. You become closed to the idea of change.

Have you ever asked yourself, "How could I be so smart but do such dumb things?" This is the effect of stress. A self-help plan must include some form of stress management, to help you let go of old habits, if it's going to succeed.

The effect of mind-body relaxation is that you don't have to work harder to improve your life. You can improve your life by letting go of the stress and negative thinking that are getting ion your way. Change isn't just about what you learn, it's also about what you let go. In Chapters 4 through 10, you will learn how to reduce your stress so that you can make room for change.

Learn New Coping Skills

There are three important coping skills for improving your life:
1. Reduce your stress and learn to relax
2. Learn to take better care of yourself
3. Let go of your negative thinking and replace it with a healthier approach

Mind-body relaxation is more than just a way to relax. It's a technique for letting go of tension and negative thinking. That's why stress management is important in self-change because you learn to let go. You let go of your fears, resentments, and the past so that you can improve your life from the inside out. If you don't let them go, what will have really changed? It is the benefit of letting go that elevates mind-body relaxation from a relaxation technique to a coping skill.

Think of it this way. There are many coping skills you need in order to be happy. If you learn them all but don't learn how to relax, you still won't be happy because when you're tense you will continue to do what's familiar and wrong.

Mind-body relaxation also teaches you how to take better care of yourself. You probably find it easier to take care of others than to be good to yourself. Poor self-care underlies every problem discussed in this book. In mind-body relaxation, you practice putting time aside to relax, which is an act of self-care. You are saying that you are worth taking time for, which begins to improve your self-care.

Cognitive therapy is a powerful technique for changing your thinking. The main idea behind cognitive therapy is that your thinking determines your quality of life. Your quality of life is not determined by external factors, but by how you interpret external factors. If you change your thinking, you will change your quality of life. In Chapters 11 through 15, I will explain how cognitive therapy works, and how to get the most out of it.

Incorporate the Changes into Your Life

All change is difficult, even good change. You have repeated your old habits thousands of times. You will have to repeat your new habits a few hundred times before they start to feel comfortable.

Both mind-body relaxation and cognitive therapy can help here. You practice being relaxed and in the moment so that you can incorporate these qualities into your life. You practice a healthier way of thinking in cognitive therapy so that it can become your new automatic response. In Chapters 16 through 30, I will explain how to use these coping skills to overcome specific challenges.

Mind-body relaxation and cognitive therapy serve the purpose of life. Combined, they help you overcome most of the problems you are likely to face. They help you identify what makes you unhappy, let it go, and replace it with something better. They transform your life.

Key Points

- Take small steps to avoid sabotaging yourself with all-or-nothing thinking.
- The most overlooked part of change is reducing your stress so that you can make room for change.
- When you are tense, you tend to do what's familiar and wrong instead of what's new and right.
- Cognitive therapy and stress management work together. They help you identify your problems, develop better alternatives, and incorporate those new habits into your life.

THE PROBLEM

STRESS AND TENSION

"Stress is the trash of modern life – we all generate it but if you don't dispose of it properly, it will pile up and overtake your life." [2] – DANZAE PACE

There are two kinds of stress. External stress is what happens around you, and internal stress, also called tension, is what you feel. Tension is your response to external stress, and it is the focus of this book.

Tension is the most important part of stress because it is what you can control. External stress is mostly unavoidable. If you have to deal with people or go to work every day, stress is all around you. The only way you can avoid external stress is by avoiding life. On the other hand, you can do something about your tension. (Most people use the terms stress, internal stress, and tension interchangeably.)

The goal of stress management is not to manage external stress, but to reduce the stress that you take on and turn into tension. If there *is* anything you can do about external stress, you'll see it more clearly and deal with it more effectively when you are relaxed.

Your ability to relax and let go of tension may be the only thing you need to change in your life. Tension destroys every aspect of life. It's hard to enjoy your life when you're rushing through it. It's hard to enjoy your relationships when you're tense or angry. Maybe there is nothing else you need to change. Maybe your tension is turning a perfectly good life into a perfectly miserable one.

The Four Basic Causes of Tension

You make yourself tense in one of four ways:
- Not being in the moment
- Resentments
- Fears
- Trying to control things you can't control

All the internal stress you feel is due to one or more of the above causes. Guilt, for example, is due to dwelling on the past, resentment, and fear. Everyone responds to stress differently. Some people let it go easily, while others internalize it. Each stress is also different. Some stresses you can deal with easily, while others are more difficult until you develop better coping skills.

Not Being in the Moment

When you're not in the moment, you're either dwelling on the past or worrying about the future. You replay events from the past again and again. You hang on to them and dwell on them. You tell yourself that you want to understand what happened so that you won't let it happen again. But how many times do you have to go over the same thing? Most of the time you're just spinning your wheels.

Understanding the past is important because it helps you understand how you got here. But dwelling on the past beyond that point doesn't help. If anything, it makes you more tense.

The time you spend worrying about the future is usually just as unproductive. Most of the time you worry about things that will never happen. Has this ever happened to you? You have a big event coming up and you worry about it and obsess over it, and when the event finally arrives you're so exhausted that you don't enjoy it or perform your best. There is a big difference between preparing for the future and worrying about it. Part of preparing for the future is being relaxed and in the moment when it arrives.

The other way you're not in the moment is when you're in a rush to do many things at once, but don't enjoy what you do. You overbook your life thinking you can relax later. But the moment you finish one thing you rush to start the next.

It feels like you're never doing enough. At the end of the day, you may have accomplished a lot, but you're so exhausted that you can't enjoy what you've accomplished. When you're not in the moment, it feels like you're surviving life instead of living it.

In the moment is where you are most happy and content. Think back to a time when you were having fun. You were probably in the moment. In the moment is where you are when you're on holiday. It's one of the things that you like about being on holiday – the chance to slow down and enjoy your life. But how much time do you spend in the moment during your day-to-day life? Learning to be in the moment is one of the best places to start if you want to improve your quality of life.

Resentments

Resentments are usually about people, and your deepest resentments are usually about the people closest to you. It has been said that resentments are like drinking poison and hoping that the other person will get hurt. The more you dwell on your resentments, the more you poison yourself, and the more the other person wins. The other person has moved on. They've long forgotten what happened between the two of you. But you're still poisoning yourself.

One thing I've learned from practicing medicine is that everyone has resentments, and everyone has fantasies of revenge. Part of the time you spend dwelling on the past, you spend dwelling on your resentments. You fantasize about what you'll say to the other person and how they'll apologize. You practice your victory address.

When I tell audiences, "Your deepest resentments are about the people closest to you," people look around as if I've exposed a deep secret. Relax, we are all alike. Even someone as enlightened as the Dalai Lama admits, "We have all been responsible for countless ill deeds of body, speech, and mind, motivated by the desire to do harm."[3]

We hold on to resentments as if they're precious possessions, instead of letting them go like the poison they are. Resentment is just another word for anger. A small resentment in the morning has the power to spoil your whole day. A deep resentment from the past can upset you years later. You've probably met people who've held on to their resentments their whole life only to end up bitter old people. What do all those resentments accomplish?

Letting go of resentments is not the same as forgiving the other person. You don't have to forgive the other person if you don't want to. Let go of your resentments because it's good for you. Let them go, because if you don't, you will continue to poison yourself, and they will become part of the baggage you carry.

Letting go of resentments is not the same as denial. Denial is pretending that nothing happened. It's an exhausting strategy because it takes work to deny reality. The more you pretend that something doesn't bother you, the more it eats you up. When you try to deal with resentments by denying them, you give them more room to grow. (In later chapters you will see how to let go of resentments.)

Being judgmental is a subtle and important form of resentment. Judgments are different from other resentments because they're so easy to justify. Your way is the right way, and the other person is wrong. But no matter how right you might be, the end result of being judgmental is still the same. You are poisoning yourself with resentments.

When you see the world as right or wrong, good or bad, you tend to focus on what is wrong. Not being judgmental doesn't mean that you agree with the other person. It means you don't want to spend your energy on things that you can't control.

One of my patients told me a sad but funny story about resentments. Gerry's wake-up call that he was too judgmental came while he was driving his son to baseball practice. Gerry was full of road rage. On this day, his six-year-old son turned to Gerry and said, "We hate everybody in front of us, don't we Dad?"

Fears

What is the most common fear people have? Most people would say fear of death or fear of failure. But if you were really honest, you'd realize it's the fear of being judged or criticized. You worry about what other people think about you. You worry if they like you, or if they think you're a failure. It affects everything you do. It affects everything from what you say to the clothes you wear.

Fear of criticism begins early with the negative criticism you hear growing up. "Don't be silly." "Can't you do anything right?" "You'll never amount to anything." "Don't be stupid." Everyone has heard those criticisms before. Small doses are normal. Parents do the best they can, and nobody is perfect. But the more you're criticized, the more you begin to believe it, until eventually it damages your self-esteem.

There is no easy antidote for negative criticism. Praise doesn't erase the sting of criticism. Being told you are loved does not undo being told you are stupid. "I love you, but don't be stupid." If you're like most people, you've probably heard both messages. The result is that you're probably an uncomfortable mix of self-confidence and low self-esteem. You're confident in some part of your life, but full of self-doubt in the rest.

Consider the case of Jennifer, a lawyer who grew up with an alcoholic father. Jennifer's dad was the nicest person in the world when he was sober, but when he was drunk he was mean and sarcastic. Jennifer can still remember his put-downs. The result is that no matter how successful she becomes, Jennifer feels like a fraud inside. On her worst days, she can still hear her father's voice telling her that she will never amount to anything.

Jennifer is successful and attractive, but she has been unable to get out of an unhealthy and destructive relationship that's been going on for years. She worries that if she was in a real relationship the other person would discover she is a fraud.

The solution is to learn how to relax. Relaxation cannot erase the past, and it cannot erase the memories of past criticisms. But it can help you let go of the doubt, or shame, or fear that you feel when memories of the past bubble up, which is the next best thing.

Trying to Control Things That You Can't Control

What do you try to control the most? The actions of other people. You know you can't control other people, but the more tense you are, the more you try to control them.

What do you do when you're standing in line? You probably try to control how fast the people ahead of you move. What do you do when you're driving? You probably try to control how fast the other drivers drive. They're either going too fast or too slow. It's crazy, but that's what people do.

When you are tense, you blur the line between what happens around you and what you feel inside. When you're tense, it feels as if things are happening to you instead of happening around you. Therefore you try to control them. It feels like people are going out of their way to irritate. But when you're relaxed, you see things as simply happening, which makes it easier to let them go.

Learning to relax doesn't make you passive. It is efficient. Mind-body relaxation doesn't involve letting go of what's important. You learn how to let go of what's holding you back.

Sounds are a good test of how controlling you are. When you try to relax, you'll be distracted by all kinds of sounds: trucks driving by, kids playing, or people working outside. Those sounds will trigger all kinds of emotions including resentment, fear, and the impulse to control.

Simple sounds become irritating noise when you're tense. Your reaction to noise is to wish it away or try to control it. You'll demonize the people making the noise, or think that they're being inconsiderate. You may think that they enjoy disturbing you, even though they don't know you are there. I can assure you most people think like that.

How you deal with the few sounds beyond your control during a relaxation session is how you deal with the many things beyond

your control in the rest of your life. If you dwell on the details of the sound, you'll only make yourself more tense. If you demonize the people making the sounds, you'll end up poisoning yourself. You will only relax when you acknowledge that you make yourself tense.

People make pilgrimages to India only to discover that they have to meditate over blaring car horns and rumbling traffic. The sounds aren't directed at you. They aren't meant to harm you. Let go of your desire to control the things you can't control, and you will be more efficient and happier in life.

There is a beautiful proverb about letting go by the eighth-century sage Santideva.[4] He said that if you walk barefoot in the world, there are many sticks and stones that will hurt your feet. Can you cover the earth with leather so that it is soft wherever you go? Of course not. But you can cover your feet with leather, which amounts to the same thing and is easier to do. Likewise, there are many things in life that you won't like. You can't control them all. But you can let go of your resentments and your desire to control them, which has the same effect and will bring you peace.

Layers of Tension

When you don't know how to relax, you build layers of tension. Every day you add more layers to the pile. Those layers damage your life because they make you overreact to things. Each layer is connected with every other layer, so that one event can trigger deeper layers.

For example, when some small thing happens, you overreact. Why? Not because of the little thing that just happened, but because of all the things it represents that you have never let go. When somebody bullies you or embarrasses you, it reminds you of all the times it happened in the past.

Consider the layers of tension you build during your average day. You may start off with a small resentment that you develop on your way to work. Perhaps someone is rude to you or cuts you off. If you don't let that go, the next resentment will build on top of the first. Once you have two resentments, you won't think of them as individual resentments. You'll just know that you're angry, and you won't even know why.

If a third resentment comes along, you'll be well on your way to taking them home with you and letting your tension ruin your evening. It's that easy. You've probably had three resentments by the time you've had lunch. What chance do you have to be happy, if you don't let that stuff go?

Tension has deep roots. Your layers of tension go all the way back to your childhood. I've never met anyone whose behavior wasn't affected by the tension they developed in their early days.

When someone criticizes you or embarrasses you, you immediately remember how it felt to be criticized or embarrassed as a child. The more tense you are, the closer those layers of tension are to the surface and the more they affect your life.

Be prepared for the fact that your layers of tension won't be pretty. During a typical relaxation session, don't be surprised to find long-forgotten resentments, sitting next to lists of worries, mixed in with embarrassments, all fueled by fear, guilt, regret, and hatred. The more you look at your tension, the more you have to wonder why it's renting space in your head.

Learning to relax changes the way you interpret the world. Tension isn't about what happens to you – it's about what you carry with you. You are the cause of your tension, and you have the ability to let it go.

Key Points

- There are four basic causes of tension: (1) not being in the moment, (2) resentments, (3) fears, (4) trying to control things you can't control.
- When you're not in the moment, you're either dwelling on the past or worrying about the future. It feels like you're surviving life instead of living it.
- Resentments are like drinking poison and hoping that the other person will get hurt.
- The most common fear is the fear of being judged or criticized.
- You build layers of tension that gradually poison your life and distort your thinking.

3

NEGATIVE THINKING

"Men are not disturbed by things, but by the views
which they take of them." [5] – EPICTETUS

Your thinking determines your quality of life. Your quality of life is not determined by external factors, but by how you interpret them. If, for example, you interpret external factors in a negative way, you will tend to feel negative.

If you think that things have to be perfect and anything less is a failure, you are setting yourself up for trouble. If you focus on the few disappointments in your life and downplay the positives, you will be prone to anxiety, depression, and addiction.

The opposite is also true. If you change your thinking, you will improve the way you feel. This is not a naive prescription to just think happy thoughts. It's a reminder that you probably spend more time focused on the few negatives than on the many positives in your life.

Negative thinking is so powerful that it can change the course of your life. What may seem like a minor tendency can end up having a huge impact. When people say they have "issues," they usually mean that they have negative thinking.

In this chapter I will discuss the common types of negative thinking and show you how they can lead to trouble.[6] I will introduce the basic types of negative thinking and expand on them throughout the book.

10 Common Types of Negative Thinking

1. All-or-Nothing Thinking. "I have to do things perfectly because anything less is a failure." This is the most common type of negative thinking, and the biggest source of trouble.

How does it lead to anxiety? You feel anxious if you think that everything has to be perfect because you don't give yourself permission to relax or let your guard down. You're always worried about disappointing others or yourself.

It can lead to depression because when you think you have to be perfect, you feel trapped by your own high standards. You're constantly pushing yourself which can be exhausting. It can lead to addiction because it is exhausting, and when you are exhausted you may think of turning to drugs or alcohol to escape.

There are many variations of all-or-nothing thinking. "Now that this bad little thing has happened, my whole day has been ruined." It drains the joy out of life. "I set big goals for myself that I want to achieve all at once." It makes it hard to get started.

2. Disqualifying the Positives. "My life feels like one disappointment after another. Nothing goes my way. Everybody has it easier than me." This is the second most common type of negative thinking.

A variation of this is being overly judgmental. "The world is falling apart. Things aren't what they used to be. I don't know what I ever saw in this person, or what they ever saw in me. They never do anything right."

This kind of thinking can lead to depression because you're focused mainly on the negatives and why things won't get better. You dwell on things that you can't control, which makes you feel trapped.

People sometimes disqualify the positives after they've suffered a major loss such as a death or getting fired. "I don't think I'll ever be happy again. Things will never be the same."

3. Negative Self-Labeling. "I'm a failure. If people knew the real me, they wouldn't like me. I am flawed. I've made a mess of things again." This also leads to anxiety because you're worried that people will discover you're a fraud. Perhaps you compensate by always putting on a front. It can obviously lead to depression because you think that you don't deserve to be happy, which makes you less willing to try.

There is overlap among the different types of negative thinking. For example, negative self-labeling also contains all-or-nothing thinking and disqualifying the positives. But giving each type a name makes it easier to identify them.

4. Catastrophizing. "If something is going to happen, it'll probably be the worst-case scenario." This kind of thinking is self-fulfilling. If you expect the worst, you might not try as hard and end up sabotaging yourself. It often leads to paralysis. "I worry that if I try something I will fail. What if I'm not up to the task? What if I make a fool of myself?" Therefore, you don't do anything, and you end up missing out on life.

A variation of this is fortune-telling. "I know this won't work. Nothing ever works for me." It creates a vicious spiral, where you don't want to do anything because you don't see the point, which can make you feel trapped and more depressed. Most kinds of negative thinking make you feel trapped in some way.

5. Excessive Need for Approval. It's normal to partly depend on other people for your happiness. We are social creatures. But if your happiness depends too much on others, it's almost certain that you'll never get the approval you crave, which can lead to anxiety, depression, or addiction.

"I'm happy when other people like me, and I'm unhappy when people dislike me." This kind of thinking leads to unhealthy relationships and poor boundaries. It can lead to thinking such as, "I'm not good enough. If someone is upset, it's probably my fault." This puts too much responsibility for your happiness on someone else.

6. Mind Reading. "I can tell people don't like me because of the way they behave." It can lead to anxiety because you're worried about what other people think of you. It can lead to depression because you feel trapped by other people's judgments.

7. Should Statements. "People should be fair. If I'm nice to them, they should be nice back." Other should statements include: "People should sense when I'm not in a good mood and give me space. My spouse should know that I love him or her. I shouldn't have to say it all the time."

8. Disqualifying the Present. "I'll relax later. But first I have to rush to finish this." In this kind of thinking, you come last. Everything else is more important. It is an obstacle to taking care of yourself and learning new coping skills.

9. Dwelling on Past Pain. "If I dwell on why I'm unhappy and analyze what went wrong, maybe I'll feel better. If I worry enough about my problem, maybe I will feel better." This type of thinking makes you dwell on the past. But experience tells you that the more you dwell on why you're unhappy, the more tense you become.

10. Pessimism. "Life is a struggle. I don't think we were meant to be happy. I don't trust people who are happy. If something good happens in my life, I usually have to pay for it with something bad." It leads to acceptance of things as they are, which makes you ambivalent about trying to improve your life.

The Negative Triad

Negative thinking revolves around three things.[7]
- **How you see yourself.** "I am flawed. I have to do everything right. I never get a break."
- **How you see the world.** "The world is falling apart. Everyone has it better than me. People should be fair."
- **How you see your future.** "Things will never get better. I know this won't work. Life is full of disappointments. If something is going to happen, it'll probably be the worst-case scenario."

An Example of Negative Thinking

Karen is a perfectionist, who grew up in a family with high standards. If she got less than an A in school, Karen was criticized. Now Karen has two jobs, two children, and tries to keep a spotless house. She's good at her job but she's always second-guessing herself. Between the jobs and the kids, she has little time for her husband, which makes her feel guilty.

By the time I saw Karen, she felt that all the color had drained out of her life. She was exhausted and depressed. She had started to hate her job, her marriage, her life, and even her kids sometimes. She couldn't understand why she felt this way because she had been so optimistic before.

Karen was trapped by her negative thinking. First of all, her all-or-nothing thinking caused her to be hard on herself. Anything less than two jobs and a spotless house was a failure. Second, she disqualified the positives so that she couldn't see the good things in her life.

She was being sucked down into a black vortex. She started to focus on the facts that supported her negative view. She found meaning in every little disappointment, but ignored the positive signs. This made her more depressed, which led to more distorted thinking. Depression created a vicious cycle.

The origin of her negative thinking was her poor self-esteem. Because she felt badly about herself, she looked to external factors for her happiness, such as having a perfect house. But the harder she tried to improve the outside of her life, the more miserable and exhausted she became.

Karen's all-or-nothing thinking was also an obstacle to improving her life. She wanted to change everything all at once. But because she was exhausted she didn't change anything. She was suffocating under the weight of it all.

Finally, her negative thinking made her pessimistic about the future. She couldn't imagine that things would get better. She confessed to me that she was thinking of abandoning her family and starting over again.

As with all these stories, there is no simple answer. First, Karen had to see that her all-or-nothing thinking was the problem. It compelled her to do more, and she was enjoying things less. She needed to lower her expectations and make some time for herself.

With a combination of mind-body relaxation and cognitive therapy, Karen began to change her thinking. Once she started to relax and developed more realistic goals, she also became more optimistic about her future. Once she was no longer being sucked down by her depression she was able to look at the rest of her life and see if there was anything else that needed changing. Her new coping skills put her in a position to deal with her future more effectively.

Tension and Negative Thinking

Tension and negative thinking are two sides of the same coin. Tension leads to negative thinking and vice versa. For example, catastrophizing (thinking that the worst will happen) leads to fear and not being in the moment. And the reverse is also true. When you don't live in the moment, you are less efficient, which increases your chances of failure, which makes you think that the worst will happen.

Here are a few more examples. When you're angry, you are more likely to disqualify the positives. When you're fearful, you are more likely to negatively label yourself. When you dwell on the past, you are more likely to be pessimistic.

Tension and negative thinking have traditionally been treated separately. Eastern methods such as meditation have been used to treat tension. Western methods such as cognitive therapy have been used to treat negative thinking. In the coming chapters I will explain the similarities between these approaches, and show you how they are stronger when used together.

Key Points

- Your thinking determines your quality of life.
- The most common types of negative thinking are all-or-nothing thinking, disqualifying the positives, and negative self-labeling.
- If you change your thinking, you will change your life.

STRESS MANAGEMENT AND RELAXATION

4

THE KEY TO RELAXATION

Being able to relax is one of the essential coping skills of life. The problem is that it's hard to relax by just *thinking* you should relax. The more you try to relax by thinking about it, the more tense you become. It's like chasing your tail. There is a simple solution to this. In this chapter I will explain the key to relaxation. You will learn a simple technique that will help you relax anywhere.

Do not try to relax your mind. Relax your body and your mind will follow. This is the key to relaxation. Your mind and body relax as a unit. They are in constant communication. But since it's hard to relax your mind, relax your body first, and your mind will follow. It's that simple. Try this one-minute experiment.

- Sit in a chair with both feet resting comfortably on the ground. Imagine your legs and feet becoming heavy. Mentally scan the soles of your feet, and feel each point where your soles touch the ground.

- It's important that you feel your skin touching the ground. Don't try to visualize it – *feel* it. Do this for a few breaths before moving on.

- Next, imagine your whole body becoming heavy and loose. Mentally scan the points where your skin touches the chair. Feel your seat and hips.

- Do this for a few more breaths before reading further.

If you did this simple exercise, you're already breathing more slowly and feeling more relaxed. It's that reliable. What's amazing is how quickly you can relax once you know how. Over the next five chapters I will expand on this technique and explain the details of how to relax.

How the Mind Works

Where does tension come from? Tension comes from two areas of the brain, and each one produces a different kind of tension. Emotional tension comes from the upper brain, also known as the cerebral cortex or gray matter. It's where you dwell on the past or worry about the future.

Physical tension comes from the lower brain, also known as the primitive brain or limbic region. It is the source of the fight-or-flight response, which prepares your muscles to fight or run. It is also responsible for strong emotions such as fear and anger. What is remarkable about the human primitive brain is that it's almost identical to a reptile brain and has evolved little in the past 100 million years.

Because it has not evolved since the time of the dinosaurs, the primitive brain doesn't discriminate between different kinds of stress. It comes from a time when all stress was due to a physical threat. Therefore the primitive brain is wired to respond to all stress, including emotional stress, by producing physical tension and triggering the fight-or-flight response. In other words, your primitive brain turns all emotional stress into muscle tension.

Reptiles get tense for a reason, but humans can get tense over nothing. Dwelling on a past resentment is enough to get your back up. When you dwell on a resentment, the emotion starts in your upper brain. Then your lower brain senses that you're under emotional stress and automatically gets your body ready to fight or run.

Why does tension lead to more tension? Once one part of your brain is tense, it triggers tension in the other part. For example, tension in your primitive brain triggers anxiety or anger in your upper brain. This, in turn, activates your lower brain, which produces more physical tension. If you don't know how to break this cycle, it's easy to work yourself into a state of panic or rage. One of the recurring lessons in this book is how to tame the struggle between these two parts of your brain.

Why is tension an obstacle to change? When your primitive brain is in fight-or-flight mode, it's wired to do what's familiar because that's the fastest response when you're under threat. There's no time to think too much when you're being chased by a predator.

In other words, when you're tense, you tend to do what's familiar – even though it might not be the best thing in the long-run. Mind-body relaxation reduces the tension in your primitive brain so that it doesn't get in the way of your making healthy choices.

The Essentials of Relaxation

There are many relaxation techniques throughout the world. How can we separate what is essential from the inessential details? Many people who need to relax are reluctant to try because they think that techniques like meditation are mystical or unscientific. I have done my best to strip away any mystical aspects and present only the essential facts.

What is essential to relaxation is what's constant over all relaxation techniques. For example, some relaxation techniques teach you to place your left hand on top of your right when you relax, while others teach you to do the exact opposite. If how you placed your hands was essential to relaxation, there would be only one way of doing it. What is constant, and therefore essential, are a few basic elements:

- Do not try to relax your mind. Relax your body, and your mind will follow.
- Become grounded, balanced, and loose. Breathe from your abdomen, and try to gently smile.
- Become centered by turning your focus into your body and away from your tension.

- Repeat a word or phrase to help you stay focused.
- Be mindful of your tension by naming it. Don't try to analyze your tension, just name it and let it go.
- Relax for 20 to 40 minutes a day.

There are a wide variety of relaxation techniques that include these essential ingredients. They go by a variety of names including mindful meditation and mindfulness-based stress reduction. I prefer to call this technique mind-body relaxation because this describes what you're trying to achieve.

The essential components of mind-body relaxation form a cycle. You begin by relaxing your body. Once your body is relaxed, your mind will start to relax. That will give you the opportunity to see any underlying tension that's preventing you from relaxing further. The underlying tension will be some combination of not being in the moment, resentment, fear, or trying to control things you can't control. Name your tension as one of those four types so that you can recognize it more easily in the future. Finally, let go of your tension by relaxing your body, which completes the cycle. The more cycles you complete, the more layers of tension you will let go, and the more relaxed you will be.

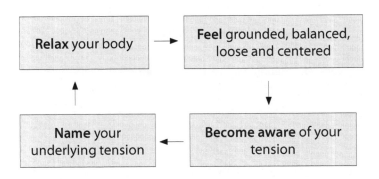

The Benefits

If you relax every day for a month, I'm confident you will feel more relaxed and happier. If you relax every day for a year, it will transform your life. These are some of the benefits of doing mind-body relaxation regularly.

- You will feel more relaxed.
- You will be able to catch your tension quickly before it has negative consequences.
- You will have less fear and anger.
- You will be more tolerant and compassionate. Little things won't bother you as much, and your relationships will improve.
- You will understand yourself and others better.
- You will improve your self-esteem.
- You will be more open to change.
- You will feel more optimistic.

For thousands of years people have used some form of mind-body relaxation to improve their health and lives. This is your chance to change your life.

Key Points

- Do not try to relax your mind. Relax your body and your mind will follow.
- Mind-body relaxation is a cycle. Relax your body, name your underlying tension, then return to relaxing your body, and complete the cycle.
- Don't try to analyze your tension. Instead, practice letting it go.
- Relax for 20 to 40 minutes a day.
- If you relax every day for a year, it will transform your life.

5

USE YOUR BODY TO RELAX YOUR MIND

There are three main areas of tension in your body. In this chapter, you will learn how to relax each particular area. The three main areas of tension are: your core muscles that control your posture, your chest muscles, and your face. In mind-body relaxation you relax each area in turn. The idea is to break the big task of relaxing your whole body into smaller ones.

Become Grounded, Balanced, Loose, and Centered

A relaxed body feels grounded, balanced, loose, and centered. Those four qualities describe how it feels to be relaxed. They are true whether you are lying down, sitting, standing, or walking. During a relaxation session, you practice producing those qualities so that you can reproduce them when you want to relax. That's how relaxation works. You practice feeling relaxed so that you can relax later.

You become grounded by feeling the contact you make with the ground. When you're tense, your body doesn't rest comfortably on the ground. You're ready to fight or run, and your muscles lift you up slightly to prepare you for what's ahead. You're, figuratively, on your toes. When you're relaxed, you rest firmly on the ground.

To become grounded, mentally scan each point where your body touches the ground, and *feel* your skin touching the ground.

Don't try to visualize it – feel it. This makes you aware of the difference between the grounded and the ungrounded parts and helps you relax. When you're very tense, concentrate on a small area that can hold your focus. Begin by scanning your toes, and work out from there.

The beauty of feeling grounded is that you can use it anywhere. If you're lying down, you can scan the points where your back touches the ground. If you're sitting, standing, or walking, you can scan the soles of your feet.

Become balanced by distributing your weight evenly. When you're tense, you're literally on edge. Your body leans to one side or the other, as if you're ready to get up and run. To become balanced, imagine the four corners of your feet, or the four corners of your seat, and shift your weight so that it's evenly distributed over each corner.

Feel free to shift during your relaxation session so that you can get into a more comfortable position. People sometimes assume that they have to sit motionless during a relaxation session. But a little moving around doesn't hurt.

Loosen your muscles. This is especially important for the muscles in your shoulders, neck, and back, where tension shows up as knotted muscles. If you have a hard time loosening your muscles, try tensing them up first. This will help you feel what you're trying to undo. Then imagine your muscles warming up or melting as they lengthen and relax.

Become Centered

Becoming centered is the most important part of relaxation. When you're centered, the center of your focus is turned inward into your body and away from distracting thoughts. When you're tense, your mind is out there, and you are thinking about someone or something else.

The easiest way to become centered is to focus on being grounded, balanced, and loose. This automatically turns your focus inward and away from your tension.

Your body exists in the moment, and when you focus on your body you connect with the moment. When you're distracted during a relaxation session, you can almost physically feel the center of your focus move out of your body and onto something else. When this happens your tension will begin to build. Do not try to relax your mind. Instead, focus on relaxing your body. Feel grounded, balanced, and loose, and you will automatically become centered again and reconnect with the moment.

To feel comfortable in your own skin, you have to be in your own skin. If you took a series of snapshots of what you focus on when you are relaxed, you would see that your focus turns inward from time to time. When you're tense, your focus is not in your own skin.

To test this idea, stop every once in a while over the next few days, and see what you are focused on. You'll see that when you're tense, it's almost as if you're not aware of your body. Your focus is elsewhere. When you're relaxed, your focus will be turned inward.

A good way to monitor whether you're centered during a relaxation session is to check what your eyes are doing. Most people like to relax with their eyes closed. When you're relaxed, you'll notice that your eyes are soft and looking forward. When you're tense, your eyes are vigilant, looking off to the side, or following thoughts in your mind's eye.

One of my favorite techniques for becoming centered is a visualization technique that's taught to cancer patients. Imagine that your body is full of white light. Scan each part of your body and imagine it filling up with white light. Cancer patients use this technique to overcome the nausea of radiation or chemotherapy. The white light represents positive emotions such as healing.

The technique helps you become centered because when you scan your body and imagine it filling up with white light, you turn your focus inward and away from your tension. I especially like this technique because you can combine it with other methods.

Breathe From Your Abdomen

Breathing is the only bodily function that you can do in two completely different ways. You can breathe either from your chest, when you're active and need lots of oxygen, or you can breathe from your abdomen, when you're resting and need less oxygen.

Each type of breathing uses different muscles and affects your relaxation differently. The muscles in your rib cage are good for producing maximum strength, but they don't relax easily. Your diaphragm relaxes easily, but doesn't build a lot of strength.

Although the muscles in your rib cage are small, there are a lot of them, and when you overuse them, they can build a lot of tension. In fact, your chest muscles are the second-largest store of tension in your body, next to your core muscles. Breathing from your abdomen allows these muscles to relax, which helps your mind relax.

Children naturally breathe from their abdomens, but most adults have forgotten how. Therefore it's worth taking a moment to describe how it's done. To take in a breath, you push out your abdomen and breathe in at the same time. This draws down your diaphragm, which opens up your lungs and pulls in air. To exhale, let your abdomen relax. This lets your abdomen sinks back in, pushes up your diaphragm, and forces air out.

You would think that breathing would be the most natural thing in the world, but when you're focused on the mechanics of breathing, it can suddenly seem complicated. An easy way to begin abdominal breathing is to let out a deep sigh. This pushes the air out of your lungs and relaxes your chest. Now you're ready to take in a abdominal breath. By the way, don't worry that abdominal breathing will distend your abdomen. If anything, it will strengthen your muscles.

Relax Your Chest Muscles

When you breathe as if you are relaxed, you become relaxed. This is the same principle as, relax your body and your mind will follow. The easiest way to relax your chest muscles is to focus on feeling your abdomen move in and out as you breathe. Rest your hands on your navel – the area that moves the most when you breathe – and feel your abdomen move.

Feeling your abdomen move turns your focus into your body and away from your tension. Don't think about breathing; *feel* it.

Let your muscles relax between breaths. When you're tense, it's almost as if you're in a rush to get to the next breath, and your breaths become short and shallow. You'll know your muscles are relaxed if your whole abdomen moves in and out with each breath. When you're tense, only your chest or upper abdomen will move as you breathe.

Don't judge your breathing or try to control it. Some breaths will be deep, and some shallow. Don't try to force your breaths or to make them deep and even. Just feel your abdomen move, and let your breaths take care of themselves.

In the beginning, there are many things to focus on, and it can be hard to breathe naturally as you keep track of them all. It's normal to feel like you have to breathe consciously just to keep breathing. But with a little practice, you'll start to relax and your breaths will begin to flow.

If you have a hard time juggling everything, remember to focus on the most important points: feel your abdomen move in and out, and don't judge your breathing. The rest will come eventually.

Variations of Breathing Techniques

There are many ways to breathe in mind-body relaxation. The main theme is that you *feel* your breath instead of thinking about it. When you feel your breath, you turn your thoughts inward.

The most basic technique is abdominal breathing, which I just described. Another variation is called "nostril breathing," where you focus on the sensation of your breath at the tip of your nose. You're supposed to feel the air move in and out past the tip of your nose, and it should feel like you're sniffing the air.

A third variation is called "ocean breathing," often used in yoga. Here, you focus on the sensation of your breath at the back of your throat. It should feel like saying the words "Ahh-Haa" with each breath.

The advantage of abdominal breathing is that your abdomen is always moving as you breathe. If you focus on the air at the tip of your nose, there is a quiet phase at the end of each exhalation when there's little air movement. Most people find ocean breathing a little distracting.

Breathing is a metaphor for life. If you're the kind of person who tries to control things that you cannot control, both your breathing and life will be tense. If, on the other hand, you learn to let things go, both your life and your breathing will be relaxed.

Relax Your Face

Your face is the most tense part of your body. You use your face to express your emotions, and to hide them. Over time, your face builds layers of tension that aren't always flattering.

The easiest way to relax your face is with a gentle smile. A smile reaches up to your eyes and down into your jaw and soothes away the layers of tension. It doesn't have to be a big smile. A big smile is easy to fake. Just be aware of smiling, and let the relaxation permeate your face.

You have so much tension in your face that in the beginning your muscles will ache as they relax. It helps to understand that almost as much of your brain is devoted to controlling the muscles in your face as is devoted to controlling the rest of your body.

Smiling is so effective as a relaxation technique that it's sometimes used on its own. Just sit and gently smile for 10 minutes, and see how much more relaxed you feel. Smiling reminds you that the purpose of life is to be happy. Relaxation shouldn't be solemn. If you forget to smile, you'll bring to your relaxation session the very qualities you're trying to let go.

"Wrinkles should merely indicate where smiles have been." [8]
– MARK TWAIN

Basic Relaxation Tips

There are three basic relaxation postures. You can relax lying down, sitting on the floor, or sitting in a chair. No one posture is any better than the others. The key is to find a comfortable position where you feel grounded, balanced, loose, and centered.

Sitting cross-legged is probably the best known meditation posture, but also the most difficult. There's a trick that can make it easier. Sit on a firm cushion, and rest your feet off the edge of the cushion on the floor. The cushion helps to keep your back straight and relaxes your muscles. If you relax lying down, you may find it easier to bend your knees and rest the soles of your feet on the ground, which also reduces the strain on your back.

Pace yourself with your breath. When you scan your body, focus on each area for a few breaths, rather than a few seconds. Your breathing is your body's natural clock. When you pace yourself with your breath, you slow down to your body's natural rhythm.

A typical relaxation session is 20 to 40 minutes. Start with 10 minutes a day, and let your relaxation sessions grow naturally. It takes at least 20 minutes to begin to release some of the layers of tension. You can set a timer if you like, or just glance at a clock periodically. It's a matter of taste. If 20 to 40 minutes sounds like a long time, consider how much time you waste worrying or being angry on a daily basis.

It is normal to feel more anxious during the first few relaxation sessions because you're not used to being in the moment. That initial anxiety usually wears off after a few weeks. But if it persists, try reducing your relaxation time to five or 10 minutes a day, until the symptoms go away. Then increase your relaxation time gradually.

Longer relaxation sessions help you feel more relaxed. There is no upper limit to how long a relaxation session should be. Try experimenting with a one-hour relaxation session after a month, and you'll be amazed at how much more relaxed you feel.

Don't think of relaxation as a first aid kit. Think of it as a coping skill. Don't pull out relaxation only when you need it. Use it as preventive maintenance. A relaxation session is the practice of letting go of tension. Like all practice, it's best to do it when it comes easiest, instead of waiting for when you need it most.

When is the best time to relax? It depends on your schedule, and on the people in your life. Most people prefer to relax in the morning when there are fewer distractions. I prefer the morning because there's always something that seems more important later in the day.

Once you have chosen a time of day, explain to everyone at home that you want to take a little time for yourself so that you can be more relaxed and happier. Nothing disrupts a relaxation session more than worrying about being interrupted. If you have a busy household, it can be hard to find a quiet time. But if your life is that busy, you have even more need to relax. Close your eyes, breathe, and experience the benefits of mind-body relaxation.

Key Points

- When you are relaxed, you feel grounded, balanced, loose, and centered.
- During a relaxation session, you practice feeling relaxed so that you can reproduce that feeling later.
- Feeling centered is the most important part. Turn your focus into your body, and away from your tension. To feel comfortable in your own skin, you have to be in your own skin.
- Your eyes are a good indicator if you are centered.
- When you breathe as if you are relaxed, you become relaxed.
- The typical relaxation session is 20 to 40 minutes.
- Try experimenting with a one-hour relaxation session after a month, and see how much more relaxed you feel.

6

STAYING FOCUSED

If your mind's not used to relaxing, it will do everything it can to be somewhere else when you try to relax. You'll make up lists of things to do or relive past events. This is normal. It's so common that the term "monkey mind" originated with the Buddha, who compared the human mind to a restless monkey that "grabs one branch, and then letting go seizes another."[9]

The most common misconception about relaxation is that you're supposed to empty your mind or eliminate distractions. But that's impossible. Besides, an empty mind isn't good for anything. Why would you want to achieve it during relaxation? The goal is to let go of your tension so that you can live a happier life, and there is a simple technique that can help.

Repeating a word or phrase helps you stay focused. This technique will greatly improve your ability to relax. Saying something replaces the chatter in your mind, which helps you stay in the moment. Any sound, word, or phrase will do. You can say something as simple as "Let go" silently to yourself.

The words you repeat are called focus words. In traditional meditation they are called a *mantra*, which in Sanskrit literally means "instrument of thought." Unfortunately, the word carries a lot of mystical baggage, so I'll avoid using it.

How to Use Focus Words

Repeating a word or phrase helps in two ways. First, it replaces the chatter in your mind. Second, it helps you recognize when you're not focused, because if you're not saying anything, you're probably distracted.

There are two ways you can repeat your focus words. You can either say them independently of your breath, or you can synchronize them with your breath.

The advantage of repeating your focus words independently of your breath is that you can speed up or slow down depending on how distracted you are. How quickly should you say them? As quickly as you need to stay focused, but slowly enough to feel grounded and centered. You can also vary how loudly you say your focus words. Say them loudly when you want to drown out the noise in your mind.

The alternative technique is to synchronize your words with your breath. This has the advantage of making you more aware of your breathing. The disadvantage is that you can't speed up or slow down.

It's amazing how something as simple as repeating a few words can be so difficult. You probably won't be able to repeat your focus words more than 10 or 20 times without becoming distracted. Before you know it, you'll be thinking about something else, and you won't even know how you got there. Fortunately this is one of the benefits of focus words. They help you realize when you are distracted.

Examples of Focus Words

Any sound, words, or phrase will do. These are just a few suggestions to get you started. You can repeat your goals: "Let go of tension"; "Scan your body"; "Stop feeling rushed"; "Be in the moment"; "Breathe from your abdomen"; "Let go of resentments"; "Let go of fears"; "Feel confident"; "Gently smile"; or, "Feel centered."

You can say what you're feeling. If your mind is racing, you can remind yourself, "Be in the moment." If you are resentful, you can say, "You're resentful. Let it go." Naming your feelings helps you see them more clearly.

You can repeat a pleasant sound. Two-syllable sounds develop a nice rhythm: "Let-go," "See-saw," "In-ohm." You get the idea.

Breath-counting is a traditional focusing technique with many variations. You can say "in" as you breathe in, and count "one" as you breathe out, then "two," up to "five," at which point you start from "one" again. Alternatively, you can repeat the same number several times as you exhale: "In. One, one, one. In. Two, two, two." This helps you stay more focused.

Match Your Words with the Stage of Your Relaxation

The words you repeat can reflect the stage you're at in your relaxation. You might start off by saying, "Let go. Let go." Later, when you're relaxed and can identify your tension, you might say, "That's a fear. Let it go." Later, you might remind yourself, "Enjoy the moment."

I like to start off by repeating, "Let go, let go," independently of my breath. This is the best way to settle my mind. After about 10 minutes, I begin to name my tension periodically. But even after I've begun to relax, there are times when my mind starts to race again. When that happens, I just go back to repeating "Let go" as quickly as I can.

There are CDs to help you with relaxation. They serve the same purpose as focus words, giving you something concrete to focus on. Many people find them useful in the beginning. But ultimately, you want a relaxation technique that is portable. You want to be able to relax without any props, using just your body and breathing.

There is a parable about mantras that puts all this in perspective. One day, a farmer went to a wise teacher to learn how to meditate. The teacher taught him how to meditate using "Om," the oldest known mantra. Although the farmer practiced conscientiously, he made little progress. Finally, the teacher asked him what he did for a living, and the farmer said he grazed cattle. "Very well," said the teacher. "Meditate on moo." Your mantra is only a tool.

Key Points

- Focus words replace the chatter in your mind, and help you recognize when you're distracted.
- Any sound, word, or phrase will do.
- If you're not saying anything, you're probably not actively relaxing.

7

MINDFULNESS

"He who knows other men is clever; he who knows himself is wise.
He who overcomes others is strong; he who
overomes himself is mighty." [10]
– Lao-Tzu

M ost people sleepwalk through life. They don't think about who they are or what they want to be, and one day they wake up and wonder why they aren't happy. If you want to improve your life, you will first have to understand how you have fallen asleep. In this chapter you'll learn how to identify your tension as part of letting it go.

Mindfulness is another word for awareness, and the two terms are often used interchangeably. The basic idea of mindfulness is that you become aware of your tension and negative thinking so that you can catch them quickly. That way you can let them go quickly. Mindfulness is an early detection system.

Three Kinds of Mindfulness

Mindfulness is usually discussed as one overall concept. But there are three kinds of mindfulness.
1. Awareness of your tension.
2. Awareness of using your body to relax your mind.
3. Awareness of being in the moment.

In this chapter, I'll discuss the first type of mindfulness, since I have already mentioned the other two in previous chapters. In traditional meditation, mindfulness means something slightly different. There the focus is on being aware of all your thoughts and emotions, and observing them without judging or analyzing them. The focus here is not just to observe your tension, but to be aware of relaxing your body and enjoying the moment. Both variations of mindfulness ultimately have the same goal: to relax your body and mind.

Recognize That You Are Tense

Recognizing that you are tense is harder than you might think. You have spent much of your life ignoring or denying it, and it won't be easy to see in the beginning. The easiest way to recognize whether you are tense is to look for indirect signs of tension, especially how easily distracted you are.

You will be distracted when tension rises to the surface and triggers a conscious thought. For example, you'll be distracted when fears or resentments bubble to the surface and you suddenly become aware of them. In the beginning, you'll be distracted so often that you'll wonder whether you're doing something wrong, or if you can relax. Distractions are a normal part of relaxation. In fact, it's normal to be distracted every few breaths.

The most common cause of distraction is not being in the moment. You'll replay events from the past, or jump from thought to racing thought. You're so used to not being in the moment that your mind will do everything it can to be somewhere else.

You'll know you're not in the moment if you're in a rush to relax. It sounds silly on paper, but here's how it can happen. As you try to relax, you'll think about all the other things you have to do, and without even knowing it, you'll be in a rush to relax. You won't think it exactly. You'll just start going through the motions of your relaxation. When this happens, ask yourself: What am I trying to accomplish? Do I want to *do* more things, or *enjoy* the things I do? Tension arises when you try to have it all.

Even recognizing that you're distracted can be difficult. You can have long trains of thought before you know it, and when you recognize that you're distracted, you won't know how you got there or how long you've been gone. But with a little practice, you'll learn to recognize your distractions, and with that you will begin to understand the underlying layers of your thinking.

Name the Underlying Cause of Your Tension

Psychotherapy is based on the idea that in order to deal with negative emotions, you first have to name them. Mind-body relaxation works in the same way. The first step in letting go of tension is naming it. When you're worried, say to yourself, "That's a fear. Let it go." When you are resentful, say, "You're resentful. Let it go."

It has been medically proven that you use a different part of your brain to name your tension than you do to dwell on it.[11] When you name your tension, you externalize it and separate it from all the other things you're feeling, which makes it easier to let go. You shift from being controlled by your tension to controlling it.

Naming your tension makes you mindful of it. It helps you observe your thoughts without getting caught up in them. It also helps you see the recurring themes of your negative thinking. Are you driven by fears, resentments, or not being in the moment?

Most of your distractions will be noise that comes from not being in the moment. But every once in a while, you'll be distracted by something important, an underlying fear or resentment. When this happens, stop and name your tension.

In the beginning, you may not know what to call your tension. If that's the case, try a few alternatives. For example, say, "Let go of fears," and you may recognize fears that you couldn't see before. Say, "Let go of resentments," and you may see resentments that you didn't know were there. The right words will ring true. If you've tried to name your tension and you still don't know what to call it, don't try too hard. You'll see it when you're ready.

Being relaxed makes you mindful of the role you play in your problems. On the other hand, when you are tense, it's hard to see yourself. You tend to think that your problems are someone else's fault. It's your boss or your spouse or the system who are making you unhappy, but it's hard to step back and see how you contribute to your own unhappiness.

Fear of criticism is a common cause of tension. If you have been overly criticized in the past, you are probably a perfectionist and overly critical of yourself. You will know that fear of criticism is an important cause of tension, if you judge your technique harshly as you try to relax, or if you get frustrated with your gradual progress. It's as if the person who criticized you years ago is still looking over your shoulder – but now you're doing their work for them.

How much time should you spend naming your tension? As much time as you need to become aware of your tension. But not so much that it becomes a distraction in itself.

Being mindful elevates mind-body relaxation from a relaxation technique to a coping skill. It makes you aware of your thinking patterns so that you decide how to change them. If you don't take the time to name your tension, you're receiving only half the benefits of relaxation.

Don't Dwell on Your Tension

Name your tension. Don't try to analyze it. When you name your tension, name it as one of the four basic types: not being in the moment, fears, resentments, or trying to control things you can't control. Then, let it go.

Relaxation sounds like "That's a resentment. Let it go." It doesn't sound like "I'm resentful, and this is why." Tension is not about what happened or why it happened. It's about the fact that you haven't let it go.

When you're relaxed, you'll be tempted to analyze what happened. But this is not the time. If analyzing what happened and why your tense was so helpful, you'd be relaxed by now.

Layers of Tension

In the beginning, it will be hard to see your layers of tension. You may even doubt whether you have any. You may think that you're just anxious and that there is nothing more to it. But as you relax, you may begin to see that you're anxious because you're in a rush. Still later, you may see that you're in a rush because you've always been told to hurry up. Still further, you may see that you're in a rush because you're afraid that if you slow down you'll be criticized or called lazy.

Don't go looking for tension. See what comes to the surface, name it, and let it go. If you want to dig deeper, you can do that during cognitive therapy.

There is a classic tale about letting go that involves two monks and a young woman. The monks are out for a walk when they come across the young woman standing by the side of a river. She can't get across because the bridge has been washed away. Without hesitating, one of the monks picks her up and carries her to the other side. Then the monks continue on their way. After some time, the second monk turns to his companion and says, "How could you have done that? How could you have picked her up and broken your vow of chastity? How could you have felt her soft skin against your face?" The first monk is a little surprised by his friend, and says, "I let her go back there. Why do you still carry her?"

Key Points

- Become mindful of tension by naming the underlying causes of your distractions. That helps you recognize your tension quickly in the future.
- It's normal to be distracted every few breaths.
- The most common cause of tension is not being in the moment.
- Don't try to analyze your tension. Just see what comes to the surface, name it, and let it go.
- If you relax without naming your tension, you're receiving only half the benefits of mind-body relaxation.

8

HOW RELAXATION FEELS

Zen philosophers have said that reading about how relaxation feels is like trying to understand the moon by looking at a finger pointing to the moon. The book can only point you in the right direction. Nevertheless, part of learning mind-body relaxation is understanding how it feels. In this chapter, I'll try to describe some of the ways that it does and does not feel.

Distractions

I've said this before, but it's so important I want to say it again: distractions are a normal part of relaxation. The goal of mind-body relaxation is not to eliminate distractions or to empty your mind. It is to let go of tension quickly and be in the moment.

Here's how the first 10 minutes of my relaxation session feels. I start by trying to feel grounded. Within a few breaths I'm making up lists of things to do. I realize that I'm not in the moment, and I tell myself, "Let it go. Be in the moment." I try to become grounded again. A few breaths later, a truck drives by. I think, "Just when I was starting to relax!" I mentally follow the truck as it drives away. It's making a lot of noise. I tell myself, "Let it go. Quit trying to control things that you can't control. Turn your focus inward." I loosen my jaw. Out of nowhere, a resentment pops into my head. I think of clever things I could have said. I tell myself, "Let it go. Don't poison yourself." A few breaths later, I'm back to dwelling on my resentment.

That's how it feels. And if I stopped relaxing before 10 minutes were up, I would think that relaxation was impossible. But after about 10 minutes, the distractions become less intense. They're less in my face, and easier to let go. After 20 years of practice, I still get distracted just as often as I always did. The difference is that now I can quickly recognize when I'm tense, and let it go.

You cannot control the thoughts that arise in your mind. That is one of the lessons of relaxation. You will always be distracted. But you can learn to quickly let go of the tension that you feel, which makes all the difference.

The Chinese monk Hui-neng (637–713) was the first to emphasize the importance of letting go during relaxation, as opposed to emptying one's mind. Previously, students were taught to purify or empty their minds. Hui-neng said that a person with an empty mind is no better than "a block of wood or a lump of stone."[12] He believed that our fundamental human nature is pure. Therefore the goal is to rid ourselves of the tension that gets in our way.

Balanced Focus

Relaxation requires a balance between focusing too little and too much. The paradox is that when you try too hard to relax, you end up becoming more tense. That happens because you're focused on getting to the end result, instead of being in the moment. You will know you're trying too hard if you're in a rush to relax, if you forget to smile, or if you relax without joy.

On the other hand, if you don't try hard enough to become grounded and centered, you won't be able to relax. You'll know you're not trying hard enough if you dwell on your distractions or become drowsy.

Most of the time, you will be on one side or the other of that balance. But every once in a while, you will quit struggling and let yourself into the moment.

Tension Has Many Hiding Places

There are many things to focus on in mind-body relaxation because there are many places for tension to hide. If you focus only on your breathing, your jaw may still be clenched. If you focus on your jaw, your toes may still be curled. In order to feel fully relaxed, you have to relax your whole body. A common mistake is to focus on one part of your body, usually your face, and then unconsciously build tension elsewhere.

How much time should you focus on each part of your body? I spend roughly two-thirds of the time feeling grounded and centered, and the remainder evenly divided between relaxing my breathing and my face. But this varies from day to day.

Spend several breaths on each part of your body before moving on to the next. If you jump from spot to spot, it probably means that you're in a rush to relax, and you're not in the moment.

Why do some relaxation techniques encourage you to focus on only one thing? Often it is your breath. The principle of these techniques is the same as mind-body relaxation. You turn your focus into your body and away from your tension. The difference is that these techniques are less direct. Sooner or later, you still must become grounded, balanced, loose, and centered. It's just that it happens unconsciously.

The Rhythm of a Relaxation Session

Relaxation feels like long periods of distractions, alternating with brief periods of calm. It's the opposite of what you might expect. Most people think that after a little practice, they should enter long periods of uninterrupted bliss. But the first 10 minutes of any relaxation session are full of distractions.

After about 10 minutes, you will enter a moment of pure calm. You will be completely relaxed and in the moment, and it will feel magical. In fact, it will feel so wonderful that you'll want to stop and admire it, but the minute you do, it will suddenly disappear. These moments are so brief that it's been said they feel like "Here I am, wasn't I?"[13]

What happens next is probably the most critical time in relaxation. You will enter another period of distractions. This is when most people get frustrated and give up. They try to relax their mind in the hopes of getting back to that feeling of calm and they become frustrated instead. Relaxation is two steps forward, one step back.

The key is – do not try to relax your mind. Relax your body, and your mind will follow. If you relax your body, you will start to calm down again. After roughly five to 10 minutes, you will enter the second moment of pure calm.

Each moment of calm will be a little deeper than the one before. Longer sessions are helpful because they allow you to enter deeper states of relaxation. During a 40-minute relaxation session, you will probably have four or five moments of pure calm. They're so seductive that you'll be tempted to chase after them. But if you do, you will become more tense. Eventually, you'll learn to flow with the magical moments instead of trying to control them.

Give yourself a one-hour relaxation session at least once a week. Try a one-hour relaxation session after you've been practicing for about a month. You will experience a level of calm that's hard to achieve in a shorter session. It will give you a tranquility that will filter through your whole day.

Relaxation Is Not Quiet

There's a lot of talking to yourself during mind-body relaxation. You're either repeating your focus words, naming your tension, or reminding yourself how to relax. If you're not saying anything, you're probably not relaxing.

But there's a difference between what you say during a relaxation session and the chatter that fills your mind during the day. The things you say when you try to relax are about the moment, and repeating them helps to connect you with the moment.

Sometimes you will have to stop and have a conversation with yourself. Do you want to continue feeling tense? Or do you want to take control of your life? I find I often have to remind myself, "Don't try to relax your mind." I talk myself through the steps of relaxation. "Are you scanning your body? Do you feel your skin? Are you centered?" Then once I'm on track I go back to repeating "Let go. Let go."

Relaxation Is a New Way of Being

You normally have two states in life. You're either awake and anxious, or asleep and relaxed. At high stress times, you can be anxious when you're both awake and asleep.

Mind-body relaxation shows you how to be awake and relaxed. Isn't that how you want to go through life? You want to be able to accomplish things, but still be relaxed and efficient as you accomplish them.

Relaxation shouldn't feel sleepy. If you feel sleepy during a relaxation session, you've probably turned off your mind or tried to empty your mind. When you find yourself getting drowsy, focus more actively on feeling grounded, breathe more deeply, or say your focus words more loudly. Stay awake by being active in your relaxation.

Relaxation Is Simplicity

Relaxation is simple but deep. The difficult part of relaxation is keeping it simple. As you progress, you'll be tempted to make it complicated. You'll forget about relaxing your body, and you'll try to relax your mind. You'll analyze your tension, instead of naming it and letting it go. You will add layers of complication, instead of taking them away. It's another way that relaxation is a reflection of your life. If you can keep your relaxation simple, your life will become simpler.

There is almost nothing new to learn in mind-body relaxation, only something to let go. There is nothing new to find, you are already there. Just let go of the tension that's getting in your way, and be free. Zen masters have tried to emphasize this simplicity by saying that relaxation should feel like "just sitting."

The Medical Evidence

Neuroscientists have shown that people who meditate regularly are happier than people who don't. Harvard scientists scanned the brains of 20 people who meditated regularly. It is known that the frontal part of the brain regulates emotions, and the left frontal region is associated with positive emotions. The study showed that the left frontal region was more active when participants were meditating, demonstrating that meditation feels good.[14]

A subsequent study showed something even more interesting. People who meditate regularly had more activity in the positive region both when they were meditating and when they were not. In other words, they weren't just happier while they were meditating; they were happier in general.

Richard Davidson of the University of Wisconsin took this study one step further. He scanned the brains of Tibetan monks who had been meditating for years. The activity in the positive region of their brains was off the charts, much higher than non-meditators, and significantly higher than "casual" meditators.[15]

The Magic of Mind-Body Relaxation

So far I have described the process of mind-body relaxation and how it feels. Now I would like to try and describe the pleasure of mind-body relaxation, which is just as important. When people try to describe how it feels, they often use surprisingly similar words to depict their individual experiences. Here are the most common descriptions.

Relaxation feels clear. You clear your mind of tension, and it is that clarity that allows you to feel the joy of relaxation. Tension clouds your mind, and prevents you from seeing anything other than anxiety or anger.

Relaxation feels joyful. There is a unique joy that comes from being relaxed and comfortable in your own skin. It's the peace and happiness you've been looking for.

Relaxation feels compassionate. You let go of your fears and resentments, and begin to embrace the world around you.

Relaxation feels energizing. Dwelling on the past or worrying about the future is exhausting. Mind-body relaxation frees you from the chains of tension and revitalizes you.

Relaxation feels magical. One of the defining qualities of a transcendent experience is that it is impossible to describe. You will know how relaxation feels once you've experienced it. When you have, you will know it has the power to transform your life.

Key Points

- It's normal to be distracted every few breaths. The goal of mind-body relaxation is not to eliminate distractions or to empty your mind, but to let go of tension quickly.
- Mind-body relaxation feels like brief moments of calm, interrupted by long periods of distractions.
- The most critical time is after a moment of calm when your mind starts to race again. Don't become discouraged. Don't try to relax your mind. Relaxation is two steps forward, one step back.
- You will know you're trying too hard to relax if you're in a rush to relax, if you forget to smile, or if you relax without joy.
- You will know you're not trying hard enough if you dwell on your distractions or become drowsy.

9

HOW MIND-BODY RELAXATION CHANGES YOUR LIFE

"We are what we think.
All that we are arises with our thoughts.
With our thoughts we make the world." [16] – THE BUDDHA

Mind-body relaxation is more than just a way to relax. It is a technique for changing your life. Mind-body relaxation is really a way to let go of tension and negative thinking. That's how you relax, by letting go of the tension and negative thinking that are hurting your life. In this chapter, you will learn some of the many ways that mind-body relaxation improves your life.

You Become Mindful of Your Thinking

Tension is subtle. Sometimes you don't know you're tense, you just know that everyone around you is annoying. Mind-body relaxation makes you aware of your tension so that you can catch it quickly before it does any damage. The faster you can recognize it, the faster you can let it go.

A relaxation session is a reflection of your life. What makes you tense in life will make you tense when you try to relax. If you often dwell on the past, you will be distracted by the past when you try to relax. How you do one thing is how you do everything. But normal life moves so quickly that it's hard to see your thinking. During mind-body relaxation you are in the moment so you have a chance to observe your thinking.

Unfortunately, awareness is a lesson you will have to learn many times. One moment you'll know that you're wasting your life dwelling on the past, and then 10 minutes later, you'll turn around and do exactly the same thing. But at least when you're mindful of your tension, you can catch yourself before you waste more time on it. If you're not aware of your tension, you won't see that you're wasting your life until most of it is gone.

You Practice Letting Go of Tension

Mind-body relaxation is the practice of letting go of tension and living in the moment. You practice letting go of tension during a relaxation session so that you can let it go in the rest of your life. That's how it works.

What does letting go of tension mean? It doesn't mean you'll never be tense again. Tension is unavoidable. Bad things will happen. You can't hope to eliminate tension permanently. Letting go of tension means that when something bad happens, you can let go of the tension that you feel, which is the next best thing. That way you won't add more layers to your load.

When you have a negative experience or deal with a difficult person, you can walk away from it and not let it spoil your day. You don't have to take it home with you, and let it ruin your evening. Ideally, you can let go of your tension almost immediately so that you won't waste any time on it.

A big part of letting go of tension is letting go of the past. It doesn't mean you'll never think about the past. You can't erase the past or pretend it didn't happen. But you can learn to let go of the tension that you feel when you think about the past, which is the next best thing.

The combined effect of letting go of tension and letting go of the past is enormous. If you can reduce your tension by 20 percent, the effect on your life will be huge. During a relaxation session you practice being 100 percent relaxed and in the moment so that you can be at least 20 percent relaxed in the rest of your life.

You let go of one thing by focusing on something else. If you have been unable to let go of your tension before, it's because you had nothing to hold onto. It's hard to relax by just thinking you should relax. But you can relax by focusing on the physical sensation of being grounded and centered. That turns your focus into your body, and releases you from the grip of tension. It is as simple and profound as that.

Mind-body relaxation makes you confident that you can change your thinking and your life. You practice changing them during a relaxation session. When you see that you can improve your mood and tranquility, you become confident that you can do it in the rest of your life. You realize that the ability to relax is not a talent you are born with – it's a skill that you can learn and improve.

"To gain knowledge, add something every day.
To gain wisdom, let go of something every day." [17] – LAO-TZU

You Experience Being Happy and in the Moment

Mind-body relaxation not only helps you let go of negative thoughts, it helps you cultivate positive ones. You experience being in the moment, being non-judgmental, and feeling happy. You experience those qualities so that you can reproduce them in the rest of your life.

You develop an emotional memory of how it feels to be relaxed so that you can access it later. It is not enough that you intellectually understand how to relax. When you're tense, it's easy to forget how it felt to be relaxed. When you're very tense, you're sometimes not within reach of your right mind, and you do things or say things that you regret later. Mind-body relaxation shows you how it feels to be relaxed and happy so that you can access those feelings.

I can promise you that this will happen. After you've been relaxing for a few months, you'll think that you don't need to relax every day. You'll think that you can relax on an as-needed basis, and save a little time. Everybody thinks like this. I know I did in the beginning.

Once you stop doing mind-body relaxation every day, you'll begin to lose your emotional memory, and soon your tension will start to build again. Within a few days, little things will begin to irritate you again. A few days later, you'll be back to your old self.

You don't learn how to relax. You practice being relaxed. People are able to lower their blood pressure through mind-body relaxation. But if they don't relax every day, their blood pressure starts to climb again. When you're constantly under stress, you have to work at being relaxed to stay relaxed.

Of course, you don't have to be relaxed all the time. Tension can be exciting. Sometimes you'll want to dwell on the past, worry about the future, relive your resentments, spin your wheels, or rush around and do many things at once. But there will also be times when you will want to relax. And if you don't know how to relax, you won't be able to.

You Take a Break from Tension

A relaxation session is like a mini-holiday. It gives you a break from your tension so that you can feel reenergized. One of the things you like about holidays is the chance to escape and enjoy the moment. Mind-body relaxation is a break that you can take every day. It's something you can do almost anywhere, and it is free.

Think of it this way. If something nice happens to you during the day, the rest of the day goes a little easier. Relaxation can be that thing. It can be a gift you give yourself every day.

The Indian monkey trap is a wonderful example of the importance of letting go. The trap is made from a hollow piece of bamboo that's just big enough for a monkey to slip its hand into. The trapper baits the trap by putting a piece of fruit inside the bamboo. Then he hides nearby. When he sees a monkey grab for the fruit, the trapper rushes the trap and panics the monkey.

The elegance of the trap is that the monkey isn't caught by any spring-loaded mechanism or moving parts. The monkey traps itself. When the monkey grabs the fruit, it makes a fist that is too big to slip out of the bamboo. In its panic, it cannot think to let go of the fruit and save itself.

The lesson is, when you're tense, you tend to do what's familiar and wrong. When you're relaxed, it's easier to step back and take a better approach.

You Learn Self-Care

As you will see later, poor self-care is one of the main causes of emotional problems. If you are hard on yourself or put yourself last, you will get worn down and become exhausted. When you are exhausted, you're prone to various problems, including anxiety, depression, and addiction.

Being good to yourself is not about material things. It is about taking time for yourself. It's about taking time to let go of the tension and negative thinking that accumulate during a normal day and wear you down.

The practice of mind-body relaxation is an act of self-care. You put time aside just for you. You practice enjoying the moment, instead of rushing through it. When you relax, you're saying that you're worth taking time for, which is the basis of self-esteem and self-care.

Mind-Body Relaxation and The Five Points of Change

Just to remind you, the five points of change are: (1) get ready for change; (2) identify what you need to change; (3) let go of your old habits to make room for change; (4) learn new coping skills; (5) incorporate the changes into your life.

This is how mind-body relaxation fits into these points. First, when you're relaxed, you are receptive to change. Second, mind-body relaxation helps you identify what you need to change by becoming mindful of your tension and negative thinking. Third, it makes room for change because you let go of the tension that is cluttering your mind. Fourth, you learn new coping skills, including how to take better care of yourself.

Finally, mind-body relaxation helps you incorporate these changes into your life by giving you time to practice. You practice being free of tension. You practice being in the moment. It is a transformative practice.

The Similarities Between Mind-Body Relaxation and Meditation

Mind-body relaxation combines the best of traditional meditation with modern psychology and medicine. It's a technique that is both accessible and deep. There are many similarities between mind-body relaxation and traditional meditation. Both are saying roughly the same thing, but in slightly different ways.

In meditation, the basic technique is to observe your thoughts, both positive and negative, and not follow them. In mind-body relaxation, you observe your tension by naming it, and then you let it go by focusing on relaxing your body. In meditation the goal is to be mindful of your thoughts. In mind-body relaxation the goal is to be in the moment.

The ultimate goal of both techniques is the same. You will be happier when you live in the moment. You will become enlightened when you see things as they really are, instead of through the distorted lens of tension and negative thinking.

Key Points

- You become mindful of your tension and negative thinking so you can catch them quickly before they do any damage.
- You practice letting go of tension and being in the moment so you can do it in your everyday life.
- You experience being relaxed and happy so you can access those feelings later.
- You take a break from your tension so that you feel reenergized.
- You practice taking time for yourself and being good to yourself.

10

HELPFUL HINTS

"There are thousands upon thousands of students who have practiced meditation and obtained its fruits. Do not doubt its possibilities because of the simplicity of the method." [18]
– ZEN MASTER DOGEN

When you first try to relax, you will probably have hundreds of questions. It's impossible to answer them all because everyone's relaxation style is slightly different. You just have to trust the fact that you will learn some of the finer points as you go. In this chapter, I will try to answer some of the common questions that arise.

The Two Most Common Obstacles to Relaxation

When you are tense, you will think you don't have time to relax. You'll tell yourself that a little tension is good for you, or that it defines who you are. You'll try to convince yourself that something as simple as relaxation can't possibly help.

Hard-driving personalities are initially more reluctant to relax. They think that their tension has given them an edge, or that they'll slow down without it. But tension doesn't make you think faster. It only makes you *think* you're thinking faster. When you're tense, you tend to do action without motion. The Samurai warriors were effective because they were in the moment. Not bound by tension, they were efficient and flexible.

A clear mind is not empty – it is open. A quiet mind is not passive – it is efficient. If you are reluctant to let go of your tension, you have misunderstood the goal of relaxation. Relaxation doesn't make you passive. Letting go of things you can't control isn't a sign of weakness. It's efficient.

Don't be in a rush to relax. The second most common obstacle to relaxation is being in a rush to relax. I've discussed this earlier, but it's so important and so subtle I want to mention it again. When you try to relax, you'll think about other things you have to do, and without you even knowing it, you'll be in a rush to relax. You will start to go through the motions of relaxation instead of actively relaxing. It's a simple but important point.

Problems and Frequently Asked Questions

Keep it simple. Once you've been relaxing for a few months, you will probably enter a phase when it will be more difficult to relax. This usually happens if you're no longer focused on the basics of relaxation. If that happens, go back and re-read the chapters on how to relax. Review some of the details you may have skipped the first time.

Expect to deal with the same issues repeatedly. You will encounter the same people and the same resentments over and over. You've spent a lifetime building many of these resentments. Don't expect them to go away after just a few months. Each time you relax, you'll let go of another layer of tension, and your fears and resentments will become less emotionally charged.

Don't worry about itches and aches. When you start to relax, you'll immediately be confronted with the problem of what to do about your itches and aches. Most people automatically assume that they have to sit perfectly still during relaxation. But a little movement doesn't hurt. If you try to ignore your itches and aches, you may end up becoming more tense. The trick is to continue breathing as you deal with these minor distractions because you build tension when you hold your breath.

There are many ways to relax. For example, you can relax by focusing on the light of a candle. But you still have to become grounded, balanced, loose, and centered. It's just that this will happen unconsciously. When you focus on relaxing your body, you are taking a more direct path to relaxation.

Don't spend more energy than you conserve. Relaxation conserves energy because you're not spending it on needless tension. Busy people sometimes take that newfound energy and do even more with it. They work longer hours, or sleep less, and do all the things that made them tense in the first place. See your new energy as a gift, and save it for what's important.

Increase your relaxation sessions during stressful times. Twenty to 40 minutes a day is just a guideline. During stressful times, try adding a second relaxation session so that you take better care of yourself. The problem is that when you're tense, you'll think you're too busy to relax. You'll think that you just need to work harder, and then you can go back to relaxing later. I understand that you don't always have time for a long relaxation session. But if you make a habit of trading relaxation for work, eventually it will become easy to drop it all together.

"The best is the enemy of the good."[19] Even with the best of intentions, you won't always have 20 to 40 minutes to relax every day. When you're pressed for time, you'll be tempted to skip your relaxation session and save it for when you can "do it right." If you don't have 20 minutes, try relaxing for 10 minutes a day. Don't limit your relaxation with all-or-nothing thinking.

There is a difference between being in the moment and living in the present. "Live in the present" is common advice that is impossible to follow literally. If you live in the present, you cannot plan for the future. But there is no paradox with living in the moment. You can live in the moment and still plan for the future, as long as you are fully present in what you do. If you want to plan, give yourself permission to plan. But don't spend that time worrying about all the other things you have to do.

Don't end your relaxation session abruptly. Take a few breaths to stretch at the end and gradually get back into the day. If you jump up and rush off to your day, it probably means you were never in the moment.

Business Leaders Who Meditate

In recent years, prominent business leaders have begun to meditate to deal with stress and improve their business and life skills. Here is a short list of examples.

- Bill Ford, head of Ford Motors
- Bill George, CEO of Medtronic, who says, "Out of anything, it has had the greatest impact on my career."
- Alan Lafley, CEO of Procter & Gamble
- Michael Rennie, managing partner of McKinsey, who has studied the benefits of meditation in corporations
- Robert Shapiro, CEO of Monsanto
- Michael Stephen, chairman of Aetna International
- Walter Zimmerman, energy analyst whose daily reports are followed by hundreds of institutional investors
- A former chief of England's security agency MI-5[20] (Although I'm sure there are many women business leaders who meditate, I was unable to find any articles about them.)

These leaders understand that they are more efficient and creative when they are in the moment. If they can find the time to meditate, maybe you can too.

Key Points

- A clear mind is not empty – it is open. A quiet mind is not passive – it is efficient.
- Don't be in a rush to relax.
- Twenty to 40 minutes a day is a guideline. Consider increasing your relaxation time during stressful periods.

A Summary of How to Relax

- The key to relaxation is, do not try to relax your mind. Relax your body, and your mind will follow.
- The three main areas of tension are: your core muscles, chest, and face.
- Relax your core muscles by becoming grounded, balanced, loose, and centered. Scan each point where your body touches the ground, and feel your skin touching the ground.
- Become balanced by imagining the four corners of your feet or the four corners of your seat, and distributing your weight evenly.
- When you breathe as if you are relaxed, you become relaxed. Feel your abdomen move in and out as you breathe. Don't try to control your breathing. Let your chest muscles relax between breaths.
- Relax your face muscles by gently smiling.
- Your body exists in the moment. When you focus on it, you connect with the moment.
- Feeling centered is the most important part of relaxation. Turn your focus into your body and away from your tension. It can help to imagine your body filling up with white light.
- Repeat a word or phrase to help you stay focused and recognize when you're not focused. Say "Let go. Let go" as fast as you need to replace the chatter in your mind.
- When you're distracted, name your tension and let it go. Name it as one of the four basic causes of tension: not being in the moment, resentments, fears, and trying to control things that you can't control. Don't try to analyze your tension.
- Relax for 20 to 40 minutes a day. Once a week, try relaxing for an hour.

COGNITIVE THERAPY

11

THE POWER OF COGNITIVE THERAPY

*"The greatest discovery of my generation
is that human beings can change the quality of their lives
by changing the attitudes of their minds."* [21] – WILLIAM JAMES

The idea behind cognitive therapy is that if you change your thinking you can change your life. Your thinking is not beyond your control. With a few techniques, you can change the way you think and dramatically improve the quality of your life.

Cognitive therapy was developed in the 1960s by American psychiatrist Aaron Beck. It has become one of the most commonly used forms of psychotherapy and has helped millions of people improve their lives.[22] In the following chapters, I will explain how cognitive therapy works, and how to get the most out of it.

Ask your doctor or therapist if cognitive therapy is right for you. The techniques in these chapters can complement the work you do with your doctor or therapist, but they should be used in combination with professional guidance.

An Overview of Cognitive Therapy

The basic tool of cognitive therapy is the thought record. It is a journal in which you write down your thoughts and analyze them step-by-step. A thought record works because it gives you a chance to explore your thoughts when no one is looking or judging.

There is magic in writing. You'll write down things that will surprise you. For example, you may write, "I feel flawed or imperfect." A thought record is a window into your thinking.

A thought record gives you time to analyze your thinking. You have time to reflect on your thinking *after the fact*, when you're not reacting out of fear or anger. Once you have analyzed your thinking, a thought record gives you a chance to look for alternatives. Finally, a thought record helps you incorporate your new thinking into your life. It helps you visualize how you might behave with your new thinking patterns.

There are 10 steps to a thought record. The first six are about understanding your negative thinking. The last four steps help you come up with healthier thinking and incorporate it into your life.

What should you write about? Journal about unpleasant experiences that you would like to have handled differently. Write about past or current experiences. Start with easy ones at first. Wait until you are more practiced before dealing with uncomfortable ones. If you have any doubts about what to write about, discuss your plans with your doctor or therapist. Write a thought record every day for a month, and see how it changes your thinking and your mood.

Thought Record Example

1. **The situation.** Briefly describe the situation that led to your unpleasant feelings. This will help you remember it later if you want to go back and study your notes.
    I made a mistake at work.
2. **Initial thought.** What thought first crossed your mind? This was probably a subconscious or automatic thought that you have had before.
    I feel like a failure. If people knew the real me, they wouldn't like me.

3. **Negative thinking.** Identify the negative thinking behind your initial thought. Choose one or more from the list of common types in Chapter 3.

    This is disqualifying the positives and self-labeling.

4. **Source of negative belief.** Is there a deep belief or fear driving this thinking? Can you trace your thinking back to a situation or person? Search your heart.

    I can hear the voice of my mother or father saying that I'm a failure and that I'll never amount to anything.

5. **Challenge your thinking.** Look at the evidence both for and against it. Make sure you see the whole picture.

    I'm hard on myself. I've had some successes. I don't always succeed, but I do sometimes. People have complimented me on my work. It's when I try to be perfect that I feel overwhelmed or disappointed in myself.

6. **Consider the consequences.** What are the short-term and long-term consequences if you continue to think like this? Look at the physical, psychological, professional, emotional, and spiritual consequences.

    I'm damaging my self-esteem. If I continue thinking like this, my negativity will affect my relationships and possibly my health. I'll be exhausted.

7. **Alternative thinking.** Now that you've considered the facts and the negative consequences, write down a healthier way of thinking. The previous steps of the thought record helped you understand your thinking and lower your defenses. Now you are ready to look for alternatives.

    Mistakes are part of the process. I don't have to succeed at everything. I might not succeed at this, but that doesn't mean I fail at everything. I have strengths that I have been ignoring. I can learn from my failures, and not dwell on them. I'm not gaining anything by being hard on myself.

8. **Positive belief and affirmation.** Write down a statement that reflects your healthier beliefs. Write down an affirmation that you can repeat to yourself.

I am successful in many ways.
"Grant me the serenity to accept the things I cannot change, the
courage to change the things I can, and the wisdom to know the
difference." This affirmation, also known as the Serenity Prayer
of AA, covers most situations.

9. **Action plan.** What action can you take to support your new thinking?
   I'm going to celebrate my victories, and focus on the positives.
   The next time I make a mistake, I won't dwell on the negatives.
   Instead I'll focus on what I can learn from my mistake.

10. **Improvement.** Do you feel slightly better, or more optimistic? This step reinforces the fact that if you change your thinking, you will change your mood. Gradually over time, your thinking and life will begin to improve.

A Perfect Combination

Mind-body relaxation and cognitive therapy complement each other perfectly. Each is suited to dealing with different aspects of a problem, and combined they are even stronger.

Mind-body relaxation is better for letting go of tension and negative thinking. For example, it is better for letting go of fears and resentments. It is less effective for analyzing them. You already know that dwelling on your fears and resentments is not helpful. No analysis is needed to make it any clearer. Therefore mind-body relaxation works best in situations where you already understand the problem.

Cognitive therapy is better for analyzing and understanding problems. For example, it is better for overcoming anxiety and depression. These conditions are so uncomfortable that you don't immediately see how your negative thinking can be a contributing factor. Your tendency is to look outward for external causes. Therefore cognitive therapy is better for dealing with problems where you can't see the role you play.

Variations of the Thought Record

This is an expanded version of the thought record. The traditional approach, introduced by Aaron Beck, uses a column format with specially lined paper. Each column represents a different step of the thought record, and there are usually five or six steps.[23] The disadvantage of this approach is that it is somewhat inflexible. You have to write your thoughts in columns, which may not provide you with enough room to fully explore your thinking.

I prefer the expanded version in journal format, where each step of the thought record starts a new line. This may seem like a small difference, but it has a number of advantages. You are not limited to five or six steps. This gives you the flexibility to take more steps when analyzing your thinking. It also gives you more room to write so that you can look deeper and make more lasting changes.

At the end of Chapter 15, I have provided a thought record template that you can copy for your personal use. You can also find a printable version in the supplementary website www. CognitiveTherapyGuide.org.

Key Points

- The basic idea of cognitive therapy is that your thinking determines your quality of life. If you change your thinking, you will change your life.
- The power of the thought record is that it gives you time to analyze your thinking after the fact.
- The thought record fits into the five-point plan for change. It helps you identify your negative thinking, let it go, and replace it with healthier alternatives.

IDENTIFY YOUR NEGATIVE THINKING

"Know thy self." [24] – THE ORACLE OF DELPHI

Cognitive therapy helps you identify the thought patterns that undermine your life. Over the next two chapters, I will take you through the 10 steps of a thought record, and show you how to get the most out of them. I'll skip the first two steps since they are easy to understand (describe the situation, and write down your initial thought.)

Let's begin with the third step, identifying your negative thinking. In this step, you choose one or more types of negative thinking from the list below. If you have a hard time choosing one, come back to this step later. Once you have analyzed your thinking, it should be easier to name your negative thoughts.

Ten Types of Negative Thinking

1. **All-or-Nothing Thinking.** "I have to do things perfectly because anything less is a failure. Now that this bad little thing has happened, my whole day has been ruined. I set big goals for myself that I want to achieve all at once."

2. **Disqualifying the Positives.** "My life feels like one disappointment after another. Nothing goes my way. Things aren't what

they used to be. The world is falling apart. I don't know what I ever saw in this person, or what they ever saw in me."

3. **Negative Self-Labeling.** "I'm a failure. If people knew the real me, they wouldn't like me. I am flawed."

4. **Catastrophizing.** "If something is going to happen, it'll probably be the worst-case scenario. I know this won't work."

5. **Excessive Need for Approval.** "I can only be happy when other people like me. If someone is upset, it's probably my fault."

6. **Mind Reading.** "I can tell people don't like me because of the way they behave."

7. **Should Statements.** "People should be fair."

8. **Disqualifying the Present.** "I'll relax later. But first I have to rush to finish this."

9. **Dwelling on Past Pain.** "If I dwell on why I'm unhappy and analyze what went wrong, maybe I'll feel better. If I worry enough about my problem, maybe I'll feel better."

10. **Pessimism.** "Life is a struggle. I don't think we were meant to be happy. I don't trust people who are happy. If something good happens in my life, I usually have to pay for it with something bad."

Identify the Source of Your Negative Beliefs

The fourth step of the thought record is about recognizing what's really behind your thinking. Are there deeper beliefs driving it? Where did you learn these beliefs? What was your role model?

The purpose of this step is to see that you have learned to think this way, which makes it easier to reevaluate your thinking and change it. You can unlearn your negative thinking, and learn something better.

Negative beliefs have layers, like tension. In the beginning you'll only see the surface of your thinking. But with a little practice you may discover deeper layers. For example, suppose someone asks you to do something you don't want to do. Your initial reaction might be to feel upset, but then do it anyway because you don't want to have an argument. What are the underlying beliefs behind this?

Maybe you don't like confrontation because you have bad memories of confrontations in your family. Maybe you saw minor disagreements turn into shouting matches, or the silent treatment. Maybe saying yes is your way of getting people to like you, but it makes you feel like you're being taken advantage of.

Negative beliefs are usually learned in childhood. It sounds trite, but it's true. This isn't going to be an exercise in parent-bashing. But it is true that your core beliefs are established early on.

Parents do the best they can. But sometimes they can't teach the best coping skills because they didn't learn them from *their* parents. Parents don't have to explicitly tell you their core beliefs. You pick them up and internalize them just by watching what they do.

One of the profound insights of psychotherapy is that adults often recreate the painful experiences of their childhood. If you grew up in a perfectionist household, you probably feel flawed or unlovable. If you were overly criticized as a child, you probably see the world in an all-or-nothing way. If you didn't receive enough love, you probably engage in negative self-labeling. If you grew up in a controlling household, you will probably be controlling. If one of your parents focused on the negatives in life, you probably disqualify the positives. If someone expected the worst to happen, you probably catastrophize. Negative beliefs have deep roots.

> *"Don't take life too seriously.*
> *You'll never get out alive."* – BUGS BUNNY

An Example of Negative Beliefs with Far-Reaching Consequences

Laura's father was a prominent lawyer who was loving but critical. Laura is nice to everyone at work, but she is surprisingly critical of her son. She wants him to be the best he can be so that he can take advantage of the opportunities he has been given.

Unfortunately, Laura's criticism is having the reverse effect. It's damaging her son's self-esteem to the point where his grades are declining. What started out with the best of intentions is having the opposite effect.

Laura's underlying negative belief is all-or-nothing thinking. Her son has to be the top of his class or he will have wasted his life. She learned this from her father, and now she's teaching it to her son. When her son doesn't comply, when he isn't a perfectionist, Laura is disappointed and criticizes him.

I encouraged Laura to start keeping thought records of her negative interactions, so that she could identify what was going on. When she became aware of her all-or-nothing thinking, she started to catch herself quickly in future interactions.

The thought records also let her imagine better alternatives. Her son didn't have to be perfect to be successful. She didn't have to be so hard on him. Her son had been a good student in the past. Laura knew he was a good kid. If he didn't feel so much pressure, his grades would probably improve.

Thought Record: Negative Self-Labeling

1. The situation.
   A stranger was rude to me.
2. Initial thought.
   People are rude to me because I'm weak.
3. Negative thinking.
   This is negative self-labeling.
4. Source of negative belief.
   I remember feeling bullied when I was growing up.
5. Challenge your thinking.
   People who are rude to me are usually rude to other people. People have been spontaneously nice to me. I shouldn't take one person's behavior and blow it out of proportion. Who knows what issues this person has? I'm not weak. I stand up for the things I really believe in.

6. Consider the consequences.
   If I dwell on other people's behavior, I will become a victim. I'll eat myself up, and they will have forgotten the whole thing. I will feel like a ping-pong ball, bounced around by other people's emotions.

7. Alternative thinking.
   People are rude because of their own personal issues. Those who are hurting, usually hurt others. I should see their rudeness for what it is. By not retaliating, I don't waste my energy, and I don't take on their tension.

8. Positive belief and affirmation.
   I will go into the world with tolerance and compassion. That's good for me, and it's good for the people around me.

9. Action plan.
   The next time someone is rude to me, I'm going to remember that they are tense and lashing out because of their own issues. I'm going to let it go, and get on with my life.

10. Improvement.

Exercise: Make a List of Your Fears and Resentments

This will give you a list of negative thinking patterns that you can analyze later in cognitive therapy. It doesn't have to be a complete or exhaustive list. Just write down a few of your important fears and resentments.

Don't worry if the list looks silly, or vengeful, or contrary to who you think you should be. This is normal, and exactly what it should look like. Most fears and resentments are irrational. By shining a light on your tension, you begin to let it go.

Key Points

- The most common types of negative thinking are all-or-nothing thinking, disqualifying the positives, and negative self-labeling.
- Negative beliefs have layers that usually go back to childhood.
- Most negative beliefs are about basic worries such as being weak, alone, or not likable.

13

CHANGE YOUR THINKING

"We either make ourselves miserable, or we make ourselves strong. The amount of work is the same." [25] – CARLOS CASTANEDA

In the previous chapter, you learned how to identify your negative thinking and where it came from. These represent the first four steps of the thought record. In this chapter you will learn how to write the final six steps. You will learn how to challenge your thinking and replace it with something better.

If someone tells you that your thinking is false, you might not be willing to listen. But if they point out exactly where your thinking is false, you might be more inclined to change. This is the benefit of challenging your thinking and writing down its flaws.

Questions to Challenge Your Thinking

One of the characteristics of negative thinking is that it tends to be absolute. You see it as fact, which prevents you from seeing alternatives. In the fifth step of the thought record you ask a series of questions to see if your thinking is false, and if so, how it is false.

Have you been in a similar situation before? What did you learn from it? Think of past experiences and what you can learn from them. For example, if you tend to think that the worst will happen, look at similar situations and see how they turned out.

How often does what you worry about come true? Does it come true most of the time, sometimes, or rarely? Most false thinking has an all-or-nothing component to it. When you're in the grip of negative thinking, you believe it will definitely come true.

For example, you believe that if you failed once, you will fail all the time. If one disagreement turned into an argument, they will all turn into arguments. If you were embarrassed once, you will be embarrassed every time. But experience tells you that this is not the case.

What strengths do you bring to this situation that you are overlooking? Are you labeling yourself in a way that prevents you from seeing your strengths? You may think that you'll never succeed, or that you'll never survive some setback. But when you think about it, you will see that you bring strengths to this situation.

Consider anxiety and depression. No matter how anxious you have been in the past, you have survived it. No matter how depressed you have been, things usually got better. What did you do to get through these situations? Negative thinking makes you see yourself as one-dimensional. But you have more than one dimension.

When you are not anxious or depressed, how do you deal with this situation? Think back to when you felt stronger. You probably had a different perspective on situations like this. You may have shrugged them off.

Are you looking at the whole picture? Consider all sides of the story. Negative thinking makes you disqualify facts that don't support your negative view, and focus on facts that support it. This distorts your thinking and makes you believe that things are worse than they really are. When you look at the whole picture don't take a narrow view of what it means to succeed. Look at success in terms of physical, psychological, emotional, and spiritual success.

If a friend was in the same situation, what advice would you give them? You might tell them to relax and not worry so much. You might tell them that you have faith in them and remind them that they have pulled through in the past. You might ask, "Why are you so hard on yourself?"

Does your negative thinking help you feel better? Is this type of thinking a positive influence in your life? Will more thinking like this help you feel better? By answering these tough questions you take down the barriers of denial and get ready for change.

Test Your Negative Thinking

If the above challenges don't convince you that your thinking is false or unhealthy, then test your thinking with an experiment. This is sometimes useful in more serious cases of anxiety and depression. Sometimes your negative thinking is so distorted that you can't think your way out of it; you need physical proof.

Let's suppose you think you're a failure, and you're so depressed that you can't see any alternative. Test your thinking by keeping track in a notepad of every time you succeed or partially succeed at any aspect of life.

The key to this is to make sure that you look at all your life, not just the big things. People tend to ignore those areas that are hard to quantify. Be sure to include everything. Try it for a week. If this isn't enough to convince you that you can succeed, then keep a record for a month.

At some point you should begin to see that you are able to succeed at a number of things. With this technique, you will begin to not disqualify your successes so that you can begin to change your view of yourself.

The Consequences of Negative Thinking

In the sixth step of the thought record, consider the short-term and long-term consequences of your thinking. Take inventory of what has gone wrong and what might go wrong if you continue to think this way. Seeing the consequences in black and white makes it easier to let go of your negative thinking.

Consider the example of all-or-nothing thinking, the most common type of negative thinking. All-or-nothing thinking is an obstacle to change. When you think in an all-or-nothing way, you believe that any change implies big change, therefore you resist it. You can't see the small steps, and you don't have the energy to take big steps, so you're stuck.

All-or-nothing thinking also creates unrealistic expectations of how quickly you should recover after a major setback. For example, after an episode of depression, you feel that you should bounce back immediately. That belief becomes another obstacle to recovery. Your body knows that you can't return that quickly. The opposite of all-or-nothing thinking is being gentle with yourself.

In the future, if you find yourself trapped by your negative thinking, pull out the list of negative consequences. Play the tape through of what awaits you. Then let go of your negative thinking and begin to look for healthy alternatives.

Develop Alternative Thinking

The previous steps of the thought record helped you overcome denial and lower your defenses. Now you're ready to brain storm and look for alternatives. In the seventh step, you will write down alternative ways of thinking about your issue.

Mind-body relaxation is especially useful during this step. When you're relaxed, it's easier to see the right answer. When you are free of fears and resentments, it's easier to think outside the box.

New Beliefs and Affirmations

Strengthen your new beliefs through repetition. The eighth step of the thought record involves writing down positive statements that reflect your new beliefs so that you can repeat them to yourself. Don't be quick to dismiss this suggestion. You've learned your negative beliefs through countless repetitions. You'll have to repeat your new beliefs at least a few hundred times before they start to feel natural.

You can speed up this process by repeating your new beliefs as affirmations. Write them down on sticky notes if you like, and put them somewhere you will see them. Repeat them a few times a day. Do it for a month, and I promise you will visualize your success more easily. This will also help you incorporate your new beliefs into your life.

I will skip the final two steps of the thought record (creating an action plan, noting any change in your mood) because they are easy to understand.

Cognitive Therapy for Caretakers or People-Pleasers

Caretakers are the people who take care of everybody else and usually put themselves last. They include mothers and fathers, older siblings, and children of aging parents. Caretakers do everything that's expected of them, and at the end of the day when they have nothing left to give, they crash from exhaustion. Caretakers are also called people-pleasers. It's a common scenario that often leads to anxiety, depression, or addiction.

This is an example of how cognitive therapy can help you change the negative thinking associated with being a caretaker. I'll skip the first two steps of the thought record, since they are easy to understand.

3. **Negative thinking.** There are at least three kinds of negative thinking behind caretaking. First, it involves all-or-nothing thinking. You can't relax until everything is finished. You can only relax when everyone else is relaxed and happy. There is no balance. Second, caretaking can involve negative self-labeling. You put yourself last because you don't think that you deserve to go first. Finally, caretaking may involve excessive need for approval. You sacrifice your time for others because you think you'll be happy if everyone likes you.

4. **Source of negative belief.** Caretakers are usually taught that taking care of themselves is selfish. Caretakers often come from turbulent or unpredictable families, where the main emotions

are fear or anxiety. Therefore they try to compensate as adults by controlling the external aspects of their life.

5. **Challenge your thinking.** Is being a caretaker good for you in the long run? Is it even good for other people? There is a big difference between selfishness and self-care. Selfishness is taking more than you need. Self-care is taking what you need. Caretakers usually take less than they need, which is why they're exhausted.

   There's nothing wrong with taking care of other people. Helping others feels good, and it's good for you. It's a normal part of healthy relationships. But you need some balance. You need to make some time just for you.

   Being a caretaker puts too much responsibility for your happiness on other people. You cannot make yourself happy by fixing the outside world. You can only feel relaxed if you give yourself permission to relax.

6. **Consider the consequences.** If you continue to live like this, you'll become exhausted and resentful. Eventually, you'll feel that others are taking advantage of you. You'll feel trapped by other people's expectations. Even further, your exhaustion may turn into depression, and lead to drugs or alcohol.

7. **Alternative thinking.** The way out of being a caretaker is to understand the difference between selfishness and self-care. You need to put some time aside every day just for you. That way you will have the energy to take care of others. If you don't take care of yourself, you won't have anything left for anyone else.

8. **Positive belief and affirmation.** "Self-care is not the same as selfishness. I need to put some time aside for me."

9. **Action plan.** You will have to change both yourself and the culture of your household if you're going to succeed. Start by preparing the people around you. That way, when you take time for yourself, it won't come as a surprise to them and make you feel guilty.

   Tell the people in your life that you're getting exhausted and that you need to take better care of yourself. All they have to do is give you a little time. They will either have to pick up the slack or lower their expectations.

Once you've laid the groundwork, start by doing something small for yourself, and expect that it will feel awkward at first. But you are creating some breathing room in that cramped little box you're living in. Eventually it will be easier and you won't feel as guilty. Eventually you will find a balance between taking care of others and taking care of yourself, and you will be happier for it.

Key Points

- Challenge your thinking by asking yourself a series of questions. Have you been in a similar situation before? What did you learn from it? What strengths do you bring to this situation that you are overlooking?
- Are you looking at the whole picture? If a friend was in the same situation, what advice would you give them?
- Write down affirmations that reflect your positive beliefs and repeat them to yourself to speed up the process of change.
- Self-care is not the same as selfishness. You need to put some time aside every day just for you so that you will have the energy to take care of others.

14

COMBINE COGNITIVE THERAPY WITH RELAXATION

"Life is short and no one knows what the next moment will bring.
Open your mind while you have the opportunity." [26]
– ZEN MASTER DOGEN

Mind-body relaxation and cognitive therapy represent the Eastern and Western approaches to self-help. Combined they are more powerful then when used alone. In fact, they are a perfect complement for one another. The small differences between them make them an ideal pair. Cognitive therapy is best for analyzing negative thinking, and mind-body relaxation is best for letting it go. In this chapter I will show you how to get the most out of both.

How Does Mind-Body Relaxation Help Cognitive Therapy?

Mind-body relaxation puts you in the right frame of mind for cognitive therapy. Cognitive therapy requires honesty and self-reflection, which are hard to do when you're tense. When you're relaxed, you can see your negative thinking more clearly.

A relaxation session is a reflection of your life. If you disqualify the positives in your life, you will do the same when you try to relax. But in everyday life, everything happens so quickly that it's hard to recognize your negative thinking. Mind-body relaxation slows things down so that you can become mindful of your thinking and see its recurring themes.

Mind-Body Relaxation Helps You Incorporate Your New Beliefs

Mind-body relaxation can be part of your cognitive therapy action plan. During a relaxation session, you practice incorporating positive thinking into your life. For example, you practice taking care of yourself, instead of negatively self-labeling. You practice being in the moment, instead of worrying about the future and catastrophizing. You practice letting go of the things you can't control, instead of focusing on should statements. You practice your new beliefs so that you incorporate them into your everyday life.

Exercise: Obstacles to Relaxation

Those are some of the ways that mind-body relaxation helps cognitive therapy. But cognitive therapy also helps mind-body relaxation. It helps you recognize and overcome the obstacles to relaxation. Do a thought record on each of the following common obstacles, and come up with healthier alternatives.

- "I don't need to relax."
- "I'm pulled in so many directions. I don't have time to relax."
- "How can learning to relax change my life?"

Letting Go of the Past

Cognitive therapy represents a fundamental shift in psychotherapy. Psychotherapy used to focus on exploring an individual's past, thinking that was the key to change. The result was that people would spend years in psychotherapy, exploring their childhoods, and often make little progress.

Cognitive therapy recognizes the need to understand the past. But dwelling on the past doesn't help. If anything, it makes you more tense and unhappy. Therefore the primary focus of cognitive therapy is to let go of the past and change the way you think in the present.

Mind-body relaxation takes a similar approach. The primary focus is to let go of your tension and live in the moment. Both techniques help you recognize your negative thinking, let it go, and replace it with better thinking. They are models for self-change.

An ancient parable stresses the importance of letting go of the past instead of dwelling on it. A man is out walking with his friends when he is wounded by a poison arrow. His friends rush him to the doctor. But the man stops the doctor from treating him. He says he first wants to learn who shot him and why. What do you think would happen to this man? He would probably die before he could get the answers to his questions. But he could live, if he just stopped dwelling on why he was hurt and let go of what was hurting him.

Key Points

- Mind-body relaxation gets you in the right frame of mind to do cognitive therapy.
- It makes you mindful of your negative thinking.
- It helps you incorporate positive thinking into your life.
- Cognitive therapy helps you overcome the obstacles to doing mind-body relaxation.

15

A ONE-MONTH PROGRAM FOR CHANGE

"People need to work at learning how to live because life is so quick and sometimes it goes away too quickly." [27] – ANDY WARHOL

I hope that by now you are motivated to try the techniques in this book and apply them in your life. To that end, I have designed a one-month program to get you started.

During this month, you will be combining both cognitive therapy and mind-body relaxation. Do them at different times of day so that you won't be tempted to analyze your thoughts as you try to relax. For example, try relaxing in the morning and writing a thought record in the evening.

Write a thought record about an unpleasant experience that you would like to have handled differently. Give yourself enough time to reflect. You can write about past or current experiences. Start with easy ones at first. If you have any doubts about what to write about, discuss your plans with your doctor or therapist.

The format you use for the thought record will remain unchanged during this month. I've included a thought record template in the next chapter for easy reference. However, the format you will follow for mind-body relaxation will change as the weeks progress. This is because thinking comes easily to most people, but relaxing feels foreign, and you will need to gradually build up your skills.

Think of this as an intensive month of change. It involves some work. But I'm sure that by the end you will feel better because of it.

Week One

Start by relaxing for 10 minutes each morning. Lie down and get into a comfortable position. Straighten out your body, and rest your hands on your abdomen. Begin to repeat a word or phrase to yourself. Try saying, "Let go. Let go," independently of your breath. Say it fast enough to eliminate the chatter in your mind, but slow enough to focus on the rest of your relaxation.

Next, focus on feeling grounded, balanced, and loose. Remember to relax your body, and your mind will follow. Mentally scan your feet, back, and hips, and *feel* your skin touching the ground. Don't be in a rush. Scan each area for several breaths before moving to the next area. Every time you get distracted, remind yourself "Do not try to relax your mind." Go back to relaxing your body.

Turn your focus into your body and away from your tension. You will automatically become centered when you focus on being grounded, balanced, and loose. This is the most important part of being relaxed.

Next, focus on relaxing the muscles in your chest. Feel your abdomen move in and out as you breathe, and let your muscles relax between breaths. After several breaths, try to relax the muscles in your face by gently smiling. Spend the remaining time focused on these four things: your body, breathing, face, and focus words.

Some time after your mind-body relaxation session, write a thought record about a past or current experience. Choose an experience that is not too uncomfortable.

Week Two

Increase your relaxation time to 20 minutes a day, and introduce mindfulness into your relaxation. Every time you get distracted, name the underlying cause of your tension. Keep it simple. Name it as one of the four basic types: not being in the moment, resentments, fears, or trying to control things you cannot control.

Once you have named your tension, let it go by turning back to relaxing your body. If you have difficulty naming your tension, just say, "Let go of tension."

A relaxation session works by being a reflection of your life. Whatever makes you tense in life will make you tense as you relax. The techniques you use to let go of your tension during your relaxation session are the techniques you will use in the rest of your life.

With a longer relaxation session, you will begin to experience moments of pure calm. In a 20-minute session, you are likely to have one or two of these blissful moments. Don't chase after them. They are not the goal of mind-body relaxation. The goal is to let go of your tension and be in the moment.

Continue to write a thought record every day, and choose experiences that are not too uncomfortable.

Week Three

At this point, increase your sessions to 30 minutes a day. You won't add anything new this week. Instead you'll practice improving and enjoying your skills. There is a milestone you will likely reach during the first month. You will be able to relax, despite frequent distractions, and despite knowing that you have more layers of tension. When you do, you will slip into the moment and begin to enter deeper levels of relaxation.

Continue to write a thought record every day. Ask your doctor or therapist if you're ready to look at more intense experiences.

Week Four

Increase your mind-body relaxation sessions to 40 minutes a day. You can break it into two 20-minute sessions if necessary. Continue to write a thought record every day.

This week, you will practice applying your new skills to your life. When you're tense during the day, take a moment and name how you're making yourself tense. For example, say "That's a fear. Let it go." Or "I'm dwelling on the past. Let it go."

Once you have recognized how you are making yourself tense, remind yourself of the techniques you used during your relaxation sessions. Remind yourself that you feel best in the moment. Do not try to relax your mind. Focus on relaxing your body and becoming centered. Take a few breaths, and scan the soles of your feet. Feel your skin touching the ground. Breathe from your abdomen, and return to what you were doing.

At the end of the fourth week, give yourself a one-hour relaxation session on the weekend, and see how much more relaxed you feel.

During this week, you will also practice applying your cognitive therapy skills. Catch your negative thinking and come up with better alternatives. With practice, you'll be able to do it more easily, and with that you will make strides in changing your thinking and your life.

Going Forward

Once you have tried these techniques for a month, do a simple test to decide if they have been helpful and if you should continue. Stop doing them for a few days, and see how you feel. If they were really helping, your tension should start to rise and your mood should start to deteriorate.

Now, complete the experiment, and go back to doing mind-body relaxation and cognitive therapy daily. Make a note of how quickly your symptoms disappear.

If you decide you want to continue, how should you proceed? You will probably benefit from doing cognitive therapy periodically. Negative beliefs have many layers, and once you have peeled away a few, there are probably deeper layers still influencing your thinking.

It has taken years for you to get here. It may take a couple of years of doing cognitive therapy to fully change your thinking and develop new patterns. But you don't have to write a thought record every day. Write one if you find your mood or your thoughts slipping. Don't just mentally go through a thought records. Write it out.

Mind-body relaxation is something that you should make part of your life. You need to relax every day in order to feel relaxed and to remember how it feels to be relaxed. You need to develop an emotional memory of how it feels to be relaxed so that you can access that feeling later. This ensures that you won't slip back to your old ways.

I am convinced that if you practice mind-body relaxation and cognitive therapy regularly, they will improve your self-esteem, relationships, mood, health, and life.

Thought Record Template

This is a template for your personal thought records. A printable version is available in the supplementary website www.CognitiveTherapyGuide.org.

1. **The situation.** Briefly describe the situation that led to your unpleasant feelings.
2. **Initial thought.** What thought first crossed your mind?
3. **Negative thinking.** Identify the negative thinking behind your initial thought.
4. **Source of negative belief.** Can you trace your thinking back to a situation or person?
5. **Challenge your thinking.** Look at the evidence both for and against it.
6. **Consider the consequences.** What are the short-term and long-term consequences if you continue to think like this?
7. **Alternative thinking.** Once you've considered the facts, write down a healthier way of thinking.
8. **Positive belief and affirmation.** Write down a statement that reflects your healthier beliefs.
9. **Action plan.** What action can you take to support your new thinking?
10. **Improvement.** Do you feel slightly better or more optimistic?

LIFE

16

BEGIN WITH YOUR SELF-ESTEEM

The pursuit of happiness begins with your sense of self-worth. Before you try to change anything in your life, have a look at yourself. If you don't like who you are, you probably won't be happy with the rest of your life, no matter how good it might be.

Self-esteem is a combination of two qualities: self-efficacy and self-respect.[28] Self-efficacy is the confidence that you can face life's challenges, and that you have something worthwhile to offer. Self-respect is the confidence that you deserve to feel happy, and that other people don't have to fail in order for you to feel good about yourself.

Self- efficacy is intellectual confidence, and self-respect is emotional confidence. In this chapter you will learn the symptoms of low self-esteem and how cognitive therapy and mind-body relaxation will help you improve your self-esteem.

The Cause of Poor Self-Esteem

The main cause of poor self-esteem is destructive criticism. You know what that sounds like: "I hate it when you do that." "You think you're funny, don't you? "You'll never amount to anything." "Don't be stupid."

Small doses of destructive criticism are normal. Everyone has heard it before. But the goal of constructive criticism is to inspire change, while the effect of destructive criticism is the exact opposite. It's shaming and dismissive. It's usually an outlet for the other person's tension rather than a motivation for change.

If you've been exposed to enough destructive criticism, you will internalize it and believe it. Over time, it will erode your self-esteem. Each person responds to destructive criticism differently. How you respond to it depends on how sensitive you are and the strength of your coping skills.

The underlying emotion of poor self-esteem is fear. Destructive criticism makes you afraid that you're flawed and not up to life's challenges. It makes you wonder if you can be happy or if you deserve to be happy. You're afraid of what other people think about you, and if they like you, or think less of you.

Destructive criticism leads to negative thinking. If you have been told that you're a failure, you will tend to disqualify the positives in your life. Your reaction may be to downplay your successes because you can't believe that you are responsible for them. Destructive criticism also leads to all-or-nothing thinking. Since anything less than perfect was criticized, your reaction is to be hard on yourself and to be a perfectionist.

A Self-Esteem Test

The impact of destructive criticism is profound. If you have been exposed to enough of it, you will almost certainly have some of the following traits.

1. **Do you feel ashamed of who you are or what you feel inside?** Excessive criticism makes you feel uncomfortable in your own skin. You think that if people knew the real you, they wouldn't like you. You think that other people are happier than you, or that they have something you're missing.

2. **Do you always feel in a rush?** The most common criticism children hear is "hurry up." Children don't live on the same

timetable as adults. They're happy to be in the moment. When you are told to hurry up, the underlying message is "Don't live in the moment, your time isn't important, and you should be willing to give up your time for others." The result is that you find it hard to take time for yourself.

3. **Do you usually put yourself last?** Destructive criticism makes you feel "less than." You think you don't deserve to be good to yourself. Maybe you don't deserve to be happy. You find it hard to accept compliments. Taking time for yourself is hard because you're afraid you'll be called selfish or lazy. The result is that you are poor at self-care, which is a major cause of anxiety, depression, and addition as you will see later in this book.

4. **Do you feel as if there's someone looking over your shoulder, ready to criticize you?** "You could have done better. I expect you to be the best. Don't be lazy. Don't be stupid." Whose voice do you hear saying that? If you've been criticized excessively as a child, you live in fear of making a mistake. The result is that you have a hard time starting things or completing things because you're worried they might not live up to your high standards. If you can't do something perfectly, you don't bother trying. It can lead to procrastination.

5. **Do you have difficulty admitting your mistakes?** Do you become aggressive, sarcastic, or withdrawn when you're corrected? Destructive criticism makes the thought of hearing more criticism too much to bear. When someone tries to offer helpful advice, all you hear is that voice of destructive criticism from years ago. The result is that you don't wait to hear what other people are telling you. You go directly to what you think they're saying and react defensively. Some people respond to that fear by being quick to criticize others. You may be the first to notice other people's mistakes. If destructive criticism is all you've known, then destructive criticism of others is the easiest pattern to fall into.

Even successful people can suffer from poor self-esteem. The details are slightly different, but the symptoms are similar. Professionally successful people, either driven by talent or rebellion, overcome the paralysis of low self-esteem. But their self-image can still be damaged. The result is that they don't enjoy their success, no matter how much they achieve. Nothing ever feels enough. So they continue to work long after someone else would have stopped, hoping to fill that void.

How Poor Self-Esteem Leads to Anxiety, Depression, and Addiction

Poor self-esteem makes you worry that you are flawed and that people may discover your flaws and think less of you. That worry can infiltrate your entire life and becomes part of the background of your life. After a while, you don't even know it's there. If you have spent the first 15 years of your life being afraid of disappointing someone, you're going to be anxious as an adult. You may not even think of it as anxiety. You may just know that you're uncomfortable in your own skin.

Poor self-esteem can lead to depression. If you've been taught that you're not up to life's challenges, you will feel trapped by your own sense of inadequacy. You may feel hopeless, or think there's no point in trying, which can cause depression as you will see later. You may think that you'll never be happy.

Poor self-esteem can lead to addiction. If you feel uncomfortable in your own skin, you may turn to drugs or alcohol to escape, or as a way of fitting in. If you feel you don't deserve to be happy, you may think that drugs or alcohol are the only acceptable way of rewarding yourself. You may think that any other form of happiness is more than you deserve.

Cognitive Therapy Exercise

How do you improve your self-esteem? You can't improve your self-esteem by working harder or trying to be more perfect. This never fills the emptiness of low self-esteem. In fact, it only feeds all-or-nothing thinking. You will improve your self-esteem by letting go of the fears that undermine it.

Try the following exercise. Make a list of the fears that undermine your self-image. Do you worry about what other people think of you? Do you worry about being judged? Do you worry about not measuring up or letting people down? Are you afraid of being hurt, or abandoned, or not being loved?

Write down the origin of your fears. Did you grow up in a family that reserved affection, was overly judgmental, or hard to please? Was your family turbulent or unpredictable so that you were never sure of your environment? Did you learn your fears in school? Were your teachers overly critical?

Thought Record: Procrastination

1. The situation.
   I don't do things that I know would help me.
2. Initial thought.
   I feel overwhelmed. I feel as if I have no energy to take on a task.
3. Negative thinking.
   This is all-or-nothing thinking.
4. Source of negative belief.
   There were high expectations of me, growing up. If I made any mistake, I was criticized. Now I have this feeling of combined superiority with inferiority. I feel that I should be successful, but the next minute I don't feel I can accomplish anything.
5. Challenge your thinking.
   I see that those early criticisms were done out of the misguided belief that they would motivate me. But it's time to let them go.

All-or-nothing thinking is hurting me. I need to look for the middle ground, which is the most efficient way to work.

6. Consider the consequences.

If I continue like this I will be paralyzed by my thinking. It will get in my way, and I won't be able to do the things I need to do to change my life.

7. Alternative thinking.

Doing something less than perfect does not mean total failure. Letting go of my perfectionism will help reduce my procrastination.

8. Positive belief and affirmation.

I will be happy with less than perfection. I will look for the middle-ground alternatives.

9. Action plan.

I will start with a small task, and be happy with achieving 80 percent. I'll see how that feels. Then maybe I'll try it with something else.

How Mind-Body Relaxation Helps

Cognitive therapy on its own is sometimes not enough to overcome low self-esteem. Many intelligent people, who understand their problems, still suffer from poor self-esteem. Letting go of negative thinking is the missing step.

Mind-body relaxation works on three levels. First, it helps you identify your fears and negative thinking. You will see if fears damage your self-esteem by how they distract you when you try to relax. Do you dwell on past criticisms? Do you feel rushed? Do you feel there's someone looking over your shoulder? Are you distracted by past embarrassments?

Once you have identified your fears, mind-body relaxation helps you let them go. For example, when you start to feel rushed, tell yourself that you're not in the moment. You practice letting go of your fears. This way, when someone makes a critical remark during the day, you don't have to dwell on it, or turn it into more than it is. You can let it go because you practiced letting it go earlier.

Mind-body relaxation not only helps you let go of fears, it helps you develop a healthier self-image. You practice being comfortable in your own skin. You practice being in the moment, which is the only place you can feel happy. It's where your self-esteem is strongest because you don't have one foot stuck in the past.

Mind-body relaxation lets you practice all these things so you can gradually incorporate them into your life. Just as repeated negative messages can distort your self-esteem, repeating positive messages can repair it.

Consider the case of Andrew, who grew up with two critical parents. Although they rarely scolded him, their way of motivating him was to ignore him if he didn't live up to their expectations. This was destructive criticism through omission.

Andrew was bright, but he doubted himself. After each professional success, he would be exuberant for a few days, but then go back to doubting himself again. He coped with his emotional pain by drinking. He wondered if people could see past his facade. He wondered why his wife was still with him, or if she was having an affair. His wife was supportive and came to all his appointments, but I could tell she was losing patience.

I encouraged Andrew to practice mind-body relaxation daily, and to practice naming his fears and letting them go. I emphasized that he shouldn't try to analyze his fears. Once he named them, his goal was to let them go by relaxing his body. Within six months, both Andrew and his wife noticed an improvement. He was more comfortable in his own skin, and their relationship began to improve.

How to Prevent Poor Self-Esteem

Poor self-esteem is preventable. Criticism is a necessary part of life. Everyone makes mistakes, and everyone needs to be corrected. But criticism doesn't have to lead to poor self-esteem. Children can grow up to be happy and productive if they learn two kinds of lessons.

The first lesson is the traditional education of facts and information that are usually taught in school. The second kind of lesson is how to let go of the tension produced by the first lesson. Without learning how to let go of tension, corrections that are meant to be helpful will eventually get in the way. Corrections that are done with the best of intentions can still lead to poor self-esteem. Teaching children mind-body relaxation is a strong defense against the stresses of life.

The importance of a balance in life and education is emphasized in the complementary philosophies of China: Confucianism and Taoism.

"Confucianism...preoccupies itself with conventional knowledge, and under its auspices children are brought up so that their originally wayward and whimsical natures are made to fit the Procrustean bed of the social order.... Confucianism presides, then, over the socially necessary task of forcing the original spontaneity of life into the rigid rules of convention. The function of Taoism is to undo the inevitable damage of this discipline." [29] – ALAN W. WATTS

Key Points

- Destructive criticism leads to poor self-esteem.
- The underlying emotion of poor self-esteem is fear; fear of being flawed, of making a mistake, of being judged, of not fitting in.
- Excessive criticism can lead to all-or-nothing thinking and procrastination.
- You do not improve your self-esteem by working harder or trying to be perfect, but by letting go of the fears that undermine your self-image.

17

IMPROVE YOUR HEALTH

*"The witch doctor succeeds for the same reason
all the rest of us [doctors] succeed. Each patient carries his own
doctor inside him. They come to us not knowing that truth.
We are best when we give the doctor who resides within each
patient a chance to go to work."* [30] – ALBERT SCHWEITZER

Nowhere is the mind-body connection made clearer than in the effect of tension on the human body. Tension damages every organ and system in the body. It directly or indirectly contributes to most diseases. In this chapter you will learn how tension causes disease, and how mind-body relaxation treats and prevents disease by helping your body help itself.

The Remarkable Story of How Tension Causes Disease

Tension causes premature aging of DNA. A fascinating study compared the DNA of mothers with chronically ill children to mothers with healthy children.[31] The mothers with chronically ill children had prematurely older DNA. The implications of this are huge.

But first, how did the researchers know that the DNA was prematurely older? The lifespan of a cell is determined by a special strand of DNA called a "telomere" that caps the end of each chromosome. Each time a cell divides, part of the telomere is used up, which makes a telomere act like a molecular countdown clock. When the telomere gets below a certain length, the chromosome becomes unstable and the cell dies. The study showed that the mothers with chronically ill children had significantly shorter telomeres, or older DNA, than their matched counterparts.

This explains the diverse and devastating consequences of tension. If the cells that line your blood vessels age prematurely, you may end up with heart disease. If the cells of your immune system age prematurely, you will be more susceptible to everything from pneumonia to cancer. If the collagen cells that support your face age prematurely, your skin will lose its elasticity and wrinkle. This single factor affects your entire body.

Can reducing tension reduce disease? The answer is yes. Numerous studies have shown that relaxation can help treat a wide range of diseases, including high blood pressure, migraines, fibromyalgia, irritable bowel syndrome, psoriasis, asthma, and cardiac arrhythmias.[32] Mind-body relaxation helps your body help itself, which is the most powerful form of medicine.

When Norman Cousins, the legendary editor of *Saturday Review*, developed a serious autoimmune disease, he chose to treat it with a combination of laughter therapy and traditional medicine. He once told his physicians, "Gentlemen, I want you to know that you're looking at the darnedest healing machine that's ever been wheeled into this hospital."

He went on to write a number of books about the power of the body to cure itself and became an adjunct professor of medicine at UCLA. He wrote, "Proper health education should begin with an awareness of the magnificent resources built into the human system."[33]

The Consequences of Chronic Tension

Chronic tension exhausts your physical and mental reserves, leaving you with no buffer against disease. The worst kind of tension is chronic tension that you push to the back of your mind, which is always there but that you try to ignore. Your body isn't designed to handle that kind of stress.

The most common consequences of chronic tension are mental and emotional. You feel exhausted, disinterested, and depressed. This is what used to be called a nervous breakdown. You'll learn more about the mental consequences in later chapters. These are some of the physical consequences of chronic tension.

- **Heart**: high blood pressure and arrhythmias
- **Muscles**: neck pain, shoulder pain, and back pain
- **Head**: headaches, teeth grinding, TMJ (temporomandibular joint) pain
- **Gastrointestinal**: ulcers, irritable bowel syndrome, abdominal pain, bloating, and discomfort
- **Skin**: rashes, eczema, psoriasis

Below are some studies that prove that mind-body relaxation treats and prevents disease. They have all been published in well-respected medical journals, and have been subject to peer-review.

Reduce the Risk of Heart Disease

Mind-body relaxation can reduce the risk of heart disease. A study in the *British Medical Journal* looked at 192 men and women.[34] The participants were randomly divided into two groups. Both groups were given information on lowering blood pressure, reducing animal fats, and stopping smoking. One group was also given an eight-week course on relaxation.

At the end of eight weeks, the relaxation group had significantly lower blood pressure. But what was more amazing was that after eight months, that group continued to have lower blood pressure. Four years later, not only did they have lower blood pressure, they also had a significantly lower rate of heart disease and fatal heart attacks. Mind-body relaxation can help reduce the number one cause of death in the developed world.

Reverse Hardening of the Arteries

Another study, published in *Stroke,* the journal of the American Heart Association, showed that relaxation can reverse arteriosclerosis.[35] The study looked at 60 patients and measured the hardening and clogging of their arteries using ultrasound.

The patients were randomly divided into two groups. Both groups received health education, while one group was also taught how to relax. Nine months after the initial ultrasound readings, the hardening and clogging of their arteries was measured again. Amazingly, the relaxation group had actually reversed the arteriosclerosis and reduced the hardening and clogging of their arteries.

How can mind-body relaxation reverse hardening of the arteries? It can happen on many levels. Relaxation reduces stress hormones such as adrenaline and cortisol, which are known to contribute to arteriosclerosis. Relaxation also reduces blood pressure, which is a known cause of hardening of the arteries. This study shows that mind-body relaxation not only prevents but treats the biggest cause of death in the developed world.

Strengthen Your Immune System

A study at the University of Wisconsin documented the strength of the immune systems of 41 individuals by measuring their antibody response to the flu vaccine.[36] The participants were randomly divided into two groups. One group was given an eight-week relaxation course, while the control group was not. At the end of the eight-week course, both groups were given an influenza vaccine. The results showed that those who practiced relaxation had stronger immune systems.

This in itself was noteworthy. But the study also had a second part. Previous studies had shown that people who meditate regularly have more activity in the area of the brain associated with positive emotions. This study showed that individuals with the highest positive brain activity also had the strongest immune systems.

Increase Life Expectancy

Mind-body relaxation not only reduces the risk of heart disease, it also increases life expectancy. This was shown in an eight-year study published in the *American Journal of Cardiology.*[37] The study randomly divided 202 patients into two groups. Both groups received standard health education and high blood pressure treatment, while only one group was also taught how to relax.

During those eight years, the relaxation group had 30 percent fewer deaths from cardiovascular disease. But they also had 23 percent fewer deaths from all causes. To put this in perspective, a medical treatment is considered successful if it can reduce heart disease by 10 percent. To reduce heart disease by 30 percent is remarkable. To reduce overall deaths by close to 25 percent is amazing.

Pain Management

Mind-body relaxation works in the same way as morphine. There are two components to pain: physical and psychological pain. The psychological component of pain is the fear or worry of having more pain. In many cases, the psychological component causes more discomfort than the actual physical pain.[38]

Believe it or not, morphine works by relieving the psychological component of pain. It does not reduce physical pain. If you've ever had morphine, you'll know what I mean. The pain is still there, but you're so relaxed that it doesn't hurt as much. Reducing the psychological component of pain reduces the total experience of pain.

Morphine does this by releasing endorphins, which are your body's own pain relievers. Mind-body relaxation works in the same way. It also releases endorphins.[39] If you relax for 20 minutes twice a day, you'll release endorphins twice a day and may possibly reduce your need for pain medication.

How Mind-Body Relaxation Relieves Physical Pain

Consult your physician before trying this. Your doctor will want to rule out if there are any serious causes for your pain. Mind-body relaxation complements standard medical therapy, but is not meant to be used on its own. Once your doctor gives you the go-ahead, start by trying this on a minor ache.

Begin by having a standard relaxation session for at least 20 minutes. Then, select a minor ache that you would like to reduce. Focus on the physical sensation of the pain. Don't try to ignore the pain or eliminate it. That will only increase your resentment of the pain and the psychological component of pain. Feel around the edge of the ache, where it's easiest not to get overwhelmed. Focus on how the pain feels at the edges. Don't think about the pain – feel it.

If you start to get resentful or slightly overwhelmed, go back to feeling grounded and centered. When you're ready, go back to feeling the edges of the pain. Then take the next step, and imagine your muscles and ligaments in the pain area relaxing and releasing tension. Some people find it helpful to imagine white light infusing the area and gradually replacing the pain. Every time you start to get overwhelmed, go back to feeling grounded and centered.

Within 15 to 20 minutes, the pain will gradually begin to diminish and sometimes even spontaneously disappear. The first time it happens, you'll be utterly amazed. But it really works. Of course, it's easier to do with minor aches, but the principle works for most kinds of pain. Some people find this technique helpful in reducing headaches, migraines, joint aches, and backaches.

The Medical Evidence for Pain Management

Mind-body relaxation has been proven to relieve both acute and chronic pain. What's amazing is how effective it is in relieving chronic pain. Chronic pain is hard to treat using conventional medicine because the pain creates a cycle. Physical pain leads to psychological pain, which causes tension, which leads to more physical pain.

How does tension cause chronic pain? When your muscles are tense, they release chemicals called cytokines that stimulate pain nerve endings. The pain is meant as a warning signal that you should slow down and change what you're doing. But if you ignore the warning signs, your muscles will become more tense, leading to more pain, which can eventually turn into chronic pain. Numerous studies have shown that mind-body relaxation relieves pain.

One study looked at 180 patients with chronic pain. They all received standard medical treatment. Half of the group also received a 10-week course in mind-body relaxation. The results were dramatic. Almost immediately the relaxation group needed less pain medication. After 15 months, they had significantly less pain. Because they had less pain, they also suffered less depression and anxiety than the non-relaxation group.[40]

Relaxation reduces chronic low-back pain. One study looked at 36 patients with chronic low-back pain. They were randomly divided into two groups. One group received intensive physical therapy, while the other received an eight-week course in mind-body relaxation without any physical therapy. Both groups were followed for six months. At the end of six months, both had improved equally in terms of mobility and lack of pain. In other words, mind-body relaxation was equally as effective as physical therapy.[41]

Relaxation reduces the symptoms of fibromyalgia. Fibromyalgia is a chronic illness that is characterized by pain, fatigue, and sleep disturbance. It is sometimes associated with depression and chronic fatigue syndrome. Traditionally, fibromyalgia has been difficult to treat because the symptoms set up a cycle, where the pain disturbs your sleep, which leads to more pain. One study looked at 77 fibromyalgia patients and treated them with a 10-week course in mind-body relaxation. Amazingly, 51 percent of the patients experienced moderate to marked improvement in their symptoms.[42] That is virtually unheard of in most treatments of fibromyalgia.

Relaxation helps relieve a wide variety of pains. A large-scale review of 28 pain studies concluded that mind-body relaxation is an effective supplement to conventional medicine for the relief of headaches, chronic low-back pain, and cancer pain symptoms.[43]

Mind-body relaxation can help people heal quickly after an injury or accident. Back pain due to an injury or accident is especially difficult to treat unless the underlying tension is treated. Patients can go through rounds of expensive investigations, require stronger pain medication, and still not feel better. This can happen if the psychological component of pain is left untreated.

Each time the person thinks about their accident, they get angry or frustrated. The more frustrated they get, the more tension they build, which causes more pain, which can turn into a vicious cycle that leads to chronic pain.

Of course, mind-body relaxation is not the only component in the treatment of pain. But it can reduce the physical and psychological components of pain. In some cases it can prevent pain from turning into chronic pain, allowing people to heal faster and return to life sooner.

Improve Your Sleep

Poor sleep is a common complaint for many people. They either have difficulty falling asleep, or have poor quality sleep. It has even been shown that people who have poor sleep suffer from a number of health problems including obesity.[44]

There is a relaxation technique that may help. Lie in bed, relax your body, and become grounded, balanced, loose, and centered as you learned earlier in the book. But instead of being active during this relaxation, allow your mind to be passive. Don't name the underlying causes of your tension. When you're distracted, let go of your tension and return to relaxing your body.

Turn off your mind, and try to imagine a completely black screen. Slowly go through each part of your body, letting go of tension and relaxing your muscles. Gradually your mind will relax and you will drift off to a restful sleep. Your sleep will be deep because you will have relaxed both your body and mind.

Look and Feel Younger

On a more superficial note, relaxation can improve the way you look. It's known that tension causes premature aging of DNA. Therefore tension can also cause aging of collagen cells, which leads to wrinkles.

But it's not just the physical effects of aging on your skin that make you look old. Chronic tension saps your vitality, making you look and feel exhausted. The way you walk, the way you talk, your outlook on life – everything is exhausted due to chronic tension.

Aging is not just the passage of time, but the accumulation of tension. The look of chronic tension is unmistakable. It's the look you see on most people most of the time: tight lips, clenched jaw, furrowed brow, and hollow eyes. It's a look that cannot be covered up with superficial measures.

Relaxation gives you an inner and outer beauty that cannot be faked. You will look, act, and feel noticeably younger.

Key Points

- Tension causes premature aging of DNA, which leads to its diverse consequences.
- Mind-body relaxation, in conjunction with conventional medicine, has been proven to treat and prevent heart disease.
- Mind-body relaxation helps your body help itself, which is the most powerful form of medicine.

18

ENJOY BETTER RELATIONSHIPS

"The heart that loves is forever young." [45]

The world feels like a better place when you're in a good relationship. Most people want one. Unfortunately, most relationships start out beautifully, and at least half of them fail within a few years.

What role does tension play, and how does learning to relax help? The cause of most failed relationships is unresolved baggage that people bring with them. They bring fears and resentments that undermine their relationship in the present.

Tension makes it hard to show affection, and hard to receive it. It makes it hard to love and be loved. Everyone knows that good communication is essential for good relationships, but communication is exactly what you can't do when you're tense. Instead, you stick to the superficial stuff, and gradually your relationship withers.

John Gottman, a world authority on relationships, has identified the essentials of relationship success. He has boiled them down to a few basic principles that are so accurate, Dr. Gottman can predict whether a marriage will succeed or fail, with 90 percent accuracy, after studying it for only five minutes! [46]

In this chapter, I will explain these principles from the point of view of tension. How does tension hurt relationships, and how does reducing tension improve them? There's nothing new about these principles. You've heard most of them before. What's new is the role that tension plays in them.

The Principles of Healthy Relationships

Healthy couples express their affection for each other every day. Even healthy couples have occasional negative thoughts about each other. That's normal. But they make it easier to let go of those negative thoughts by expressing their affection for each other every day. That way, when negative thoughts arise, they don't overwhelm their positive feelings.

When you give and receive affection daily, it's easier to shrug off little annoyances. Hearing, "I love you," or "You look good today," makes a world of difference. Later, when one of you is a little short with the other, or when one of you speaks in a certain tone of voice, it's easier to assume that it's because the other person is tired, instead of assuming that they're angry or don't love you. Romance means celebrating the positive things in a relationship. Without those expressions of affection, it's easy for little annoyances to build into big resentments.

What role does tension play? Tension makes it hard to let go of negative thoughts. You tend to focus on the negatives and dwell on the past. Mind-body relaxation prevents small things from getting in the way of important things, like saying "I love you."

Healthy couples acknowledge each other's invitations for affection. Every day, your partner makes small overtures for your affection. They offer bits of conversation, or enter your physical space hoping for a hug. It's one of the ways that healthy couples strengthen the bond between each other.

That is hard to do when you're tense. Those gentle invitations are usually bits of conversation. Nothing important. In fact they're not meant to be important. They're just an opening for something bigger – a hug or a kiss. But when you're tense, you tend to take those gentle invitations literally, and ignore them or criticize them.

You can't see past their smallness to what they really mean – "Please give me a hug."

Healthy couples show respect for each other by asking the other's opinion, and following it when it has merit. When you're tense, it's hard to be open to someone else's opinion. You have one way of seeing things and one way of doing things – your way. Even if it's the wrong way, you stick with what you know out of stubbornness and because there isn't room in a tense mind for anything else.

Healthy couples offer conciliatory gestures to prevent disagreements from escalating. Healthy couples disagree just as much as unhealthy ones. But they disagree differently. They don't allow their disagreements to get out of control. They make conciliatory gestures, like saying, "I'm sorry," or "Let's try that again."

Have you ever sat down hoping to have a civilized conversation, only to watch it turn into an argument? When you're tense you bring in stresses from your day, and let them contaminate your conversation. You're really angry about something that happened earlier, but you take it out on the person you love. If you're not mindful of your tension, you won't even know why you're angry, you'll just know that you are. When you're relaxed, it's easier to leave that stuff at work. You have fewer buttons to push.

Healthy couples ask what the other is thinking or feeling, and take the time to listen. Couples fear growing apart, but do little to prevent it. Knowing what your partner is thinking and feeling is one of the best protections against growing apart. It's a given that you will both grow and change over time. Healthy relationships can handle differences. What they can't handle is silence. When you're tense, you only talk about superficial stuff – if you talk at all, and with each conversation, your relationship grows more superficial.

Being in the moment helps you hear what your partner is saying. This is especially true for the subtle messages people send out in the early stages of relationship problems. When problems are still small, most people don't explicitly say there is something wrong. Instead, they send out indirect signals that can be hard to read.

Those signals are especially hard to read when you're tense. But you ignore them at your peril. They may be nothing to worry about, but they can also be a sign that you're starting to drift apart. When you're relaxed and in the moment, it's easier to sit down and hear those subtle signs and catch little problems before they turn into big ones.

Healthy couples appreciate the positives, and don't disqualify them. They tell their partner that they appreciate their positive qualities. They don't take those qualities for granted. They don't assume that their partner knows they are appreciated.

Healthy couples are kind to each other. The one word that best summarizes the above points is – kindness. When you see healthy couples, you are struck by how gentle and kind they are with each other. But kindness comes from being relaxed. Mind-body relaxation helps you practice the loving-kindness that is the basis of healthy relationships.

If you're still not sure of the importance of mind-body relaxation in your relationship, ask yourself this: will more resentments, more fears, and more stress improve your situation?

The Signs of Unhealthy Relationships

This section looks at the flip side of healthy relationships. How does tension make good relationships bad, and unhealthy relationships worse?

Unhealthy couples begin arguments harshly. They begin by detailing what's wrong, and why the other person is at fault. Research has shown that when disagreements begin in that tone, 96 percent of the time, they will end negatively, even if the couple tries to "make nice" in between.[47]

What role does tension play? When you're tense, you want to get stuff off your chest, and you're not thinking about the other person's feelings. If you've had a bad day, and your partner isn't fully supportive or if they're a little distracted, it's easy to take out your frustrations on them. You forget the real cause of your anger.

When you're relaxed, it's easier to see the big picture. Take a deep breath, and focus on what's really bothering you. Or better yet, when you come home, take 20 minutes to relax so that you can let go of your resentments and enjoy your evening.

When you have a disagreement, start by focusing on the positives. Begin with how much your relationship means to you. Don't just say the words – mean them. Remember that you're holding something fragile in your hands when you begin an argument. Begin with the positives, not only to reassure your partner, but also to remind yourself of the big picture. That's easier to do when you're relaxed.

Unhealthy couples are unkind to each other, and engage in a death spiral of criticism and contempt. It begins with criticism. Unhealthy couples don't offer suggestions. They go beyond the problem at hand and criticize their partner's character. It sounds like "Could you please clean up this mess? You're so lazy." The more tense you are, the more criticism can escalate into contempt. "You're such a slob."

Contempt is the most deadly part of the death spiral because it involves name-calling, which implies that you're disgusted with your partner. No one can have a rational conversation if they think you're disgusted with them. Once contempt is out of the bag, defensiveness soon follows. Your partner responds with why it's not their fault. "I'll clean it up eventually, but you're the one who started dinner late."

The final step is withdrawal. One or the other feels overwhelmed and stops communicating. The less one communicates, the more the other becomes agitated and contemptuous. Can you see the role that tension plays in this story? It is all driven by tension, fears, and resentments.

Unhealthy couples turn away from conciliatory gestures. Even if your relationship has all the unhealthy qualities listed above, it can still survive if it has one positive quality. Healthy couples turn toward each other after an argument. They offer conciliatory gestures to repair hurt feelings. Studies have shown that couples who turn toward each other after an argument, even if they have all the above unhealthy qualities, still have an 84 percent chance of remaining happily married.[48]

Unhealthy couples disqualify the positives and focus on the negatives. They may start out being infatuated with each other, but then they quickly focus on what is wrong with the other person, and why they're not a good match.

Eventually they may look for someone else (which usually means different from the last one). Once they have settled into their new relationship, they discover that they have to make a new set of compromises. And once again, they become dissatisfied and move on to the next relationship. When you are tense, you tend to disqualify the positives. Tension contributes to all the qualities of unhealthy relationships.

A Summary of Relationships

Unhealthy couples:

- Begin arguments harshly, with why the other person is at fault.
- Turn away from conciliatory gestures.
- Disqualify the positives and focus on the negatives.
- They are unkind to each other, and engage in a death spiral of criticism and contempt.

Healthy couples:

- Express their affection for each other every day, which helps to smooth over minor differences.
- Acknowledge each other's invitations for affection.
- Show respect for each other by asking the other's opinion, and following it when it has merit.
- Offer conciliatory gestures to prevent disagreements from escalating.
- Ask what the other is thinking or feeling, and take the time to listen.
- Appreciate the positives, and don't disqualify them.
- They are kind to each other.

Consider the case of Norman and Margaret. They both have busy careers and teenage children at home. He's a recovering alcoholic, who had been doing well for two years. In our sessions, Margaret repeatedly said she was resentful of all the things he had put her through. She was justifiably upset.

Norman had been a Jekyll and Hyde when he was drinking. He had embarrassed Margaret and had been rude to her. But these resentments were now getting in the way of their mutual recovery. They had been to couples counseling for the past two years, but made little progress. During our sessions, Margaret would sit with her arms crossed and correct every statement that Norman made.

One day, I asked Margaret what it would take for her to begin to let go of her resentments. She said she was resentful that Norman had the luxury to go to rehab and focus on himself, while she had to hold the family together. I suggested that it was Margaret's turn to take care of herself. I encouraged her to put some time aside every day to relax. Norman and the children would have to take up the slack or change their expectations. Their recovery had to be mutual.

Both Margaret and Norman had to feel better about their lives if this was going to work. Margaret took my suggestion and began to relax every day. After a few months, she felt a little better and started noticing that she was more tolerant toward her husband and children. Gradually, the barriers began to come down, and they started making progress as a couple.

Effective Communication

All effective communication is win-win. Both people have to feel they're getting something positive from communication if it's going to work. If you want to be heard and influence your partner, they will only listen if they feel they're being treated with respect. Effective communication doesn't sound like, "Let me tell you why you're wrong."

There is no win-lose communication in a relationship. If one person has to lose, they will make sure that the other person doesn't get to win in the long run. Nobody accepts being treated badly for ever. I have seen the meekest people eventually rise up and take on the person who tried to control them. In relationships, either both people win or both people lose.

But when you're tense, it's hard to think in terms of win-win. You forget about the other person's feelings because you want to make your point. You tend to see your choices as all-or-nothing. You think that if you bend a little, it will be seen as a sign of weakness.

Healthy couples don't have to agree all the time. You can disagree on issues without attacking the other person. You can offer suggestions without name-calling. But you will only do it when you're relaxed. That's when it's easier to speak with compassion, and listen with understanding. That's when you can acknowledge what the other person is saying, and stick to the issues. It's never easy. But it's a lot harder when you're tense.

Key Points

- Tension makes it hard to love and be loved.
- Tension leads to arguments, contempt, and the relationship death spiral.
- Tension makes you disqualify the positives.
- Mind-body relaxation makes it easier to show affection and accept it.
- It prevents little annoyances from turning into major resentments.
- It makes it easier to focus on the positives, and be kind to each other.

19

DEVELOP TOLERANCE
AND COMPASSION

"If possible, you should help others. If that is not possible,
at least you should do no harm." [49] – THE DALAI LAMA

Tolerance and compassion are the basis of all human relationships. All major religions are founded on them. They bring out the best in people, and help people bring out the best in each other. But they are hard to express when you're tense. In this chapter you will learn how mind-body relaxation nurtures the human soul.

Understanding

Tolerance and compassion begin with understanding. In order to understand people, you first have to understand how they deal with tension. People are driven by tension. Most people spend more time feeling anxious or angry than they do feeling joyful or happy.

There are other factors that you have to know about people of course. But if you don't understand how they deal with tension, they'll surprise you most of the time. Because when they are tense, they tend to do what's familiar, even when it's wrong.

Most of the bad behavior you encounter during the day is due to the fact that people are up to their eyeballs in tension. You say something that seems innocent, and without knowing it, you trigger some deep layer of anxiety or vulnerability. Suddenly, the other person snaps.

Mind-body relaxation helps you understand other people because it helps you understand yourself. It makes you mindful of your underlying tension, and how you respond when you are tense. Understanding will help you avoid conflicts and repair relationships.

Compassion

Compassion is the most beautiful expression of the human spirit. It is how we connect with each other. Every adult can remember someone whose compassion had a pivotal impact on their life. Children respond to the positive influence of compassion. A small gesture can sometimes turn around an adversary. You have as many reasons for compassion as you have relationships in your life.

Call it enlightened self-interest, but it's hard to like yourself when you're not compassionate. But the best reason to do the right thing is that it's the right thing for you. Anger and intolerance don't leave room in your heart for anything else, including liking yourself.

Of course, it's easy to say that we *should* be compassionate and tolerant. But how do we do that in a stressful world? This is where mind-body relaxation is especially helpful. It does not prescribe that you should be compassionate. It gives you a compass that points you in the direction of compassion and tolerance.

We are born with the capacity for compassion. As a species we could not exist without it. Therefore you don't have to learn how to be compassionate. You just have to let go of the tension that is getting in your way. If you practice relaxation every day, you will become more compassionate.

Compassion is not that hard to understand. It is just another word for kindness. The Dalai Lama writes, "My religion is kindness."[50] When your mind is clear of tension and your heart is free of fears and resentments, you will find the compassion within you.

Tolerance

Compassion is always the best approach, but sometimes that's not always possible. Every day you will meet angry and insensitive people who are living under extraordinary stress. Sometimes the best you can do is understand that they are full of tension and not get caught up in it.

Sometimes the best you can do is tolerate the other person's behavior. That doesn't mean you agree with it or condone it. It just means you realize there are some things you cannot control, and becoming angry will not help. If there is a chance you can help someone change, it's more likely to happen in a climate of tolerance.

Tolerance is preferable to anger, because tolerance is cheaper than aggression. The main victim of your anger is you. This is described eloquently in the Buddhist expression, "You will not be punished for your anger – you will be punished by your anger."[51]

Sometimes even your capacity for tolerance will be tested. Some people will push you to the limit. You've tried to set healthy boundaries, you've tried to be tolerant, but they just don't get it. They're so full of hurt and anger themselves that they can't appreciate your tolerance. In this case, the best thing you can do is avoid them, because this too is a form of tolerance.

Let Go of Deep Resentments

Part of tolerance is learning to let go of resentments. The question is not whether you have deep resentments, but what you will do with them. Will you hold on to them until the other person has apologized? Will you dwell on your fantasies of revenge until they poison you? Or will you let them go?

Let go of your resentments because it's good for you. Let go of your resentments because if you don't, you will continue to suffer. Let them go because the other person has moved on and you're still hurting yourself. Why do you tell your friends to let go of their resentments, but you continue to hold on to yours?

How do you let go of deep resentments? The same way you let go of tension. You can't permanently eliminate resentments. But you can learn to quickly let go of the resentments that you feel when you think about the past, which is the next best thing.

Don't be in a rush to let go of deep resentments. They have deep roots, and crop up when you least expect them. They are connected to your subconscious and can be triggered by almost anything. You'll be minding your own business, when all of a sudden one will pop up, and make you just as angry as it did years ago.

If you rush to let it go, if you think it's silly that you're still resentful, you'll overlook its deep roots and never completely let it go. You've been cultivating some of these resentments for years. It will take a little practice to let them go.

When you find yourself struggling to let go of a resentment, stop and give yourself a choice. You can dwell on your resentment, or let it go. You can give the other person power over you, or you take control of your life. You can poison yourself, or move on.

The Medical Evidence

Your happiness spreads like ripples in a pond, affecting the people around you.[52] This is not just motherly advice, but a proven scientific fact. When you are happier, the people who are socially close to you, such as family members, also become happier because of the ripple effect.

This effect was discovered by following almost 5,000 people over 20 years in the Framingham Heart Study social network. The study showed that happiness spreads between people over time and results in clusters of happiness. The clusters are more than just the effect of happy people seeking out other happy people and avoiding unhappy ones.

Amazingly, the effect transcends direct links and reaches a third degree of separation. When you are happier, a friend of a friend has a greater chance of being happier, despite the fact they don't know you directly.

It has been said that we live in a time of material abundance and emotional poverty. Perhaps one way to correct this is by approaching happiness as a health phenomenon that spreads from person to person. This study is a reminder that if you want to make a difference in the world, the best place to start is by working on yourself.

Key Points

- The best reason to do the right thing is that it's the right thing for you.
- You will not be punished for your anger – you will be punished by your anger.
- Mind-body relaxation gives you a compass that points you in the direction of compassion and tolerance.
- Go into the world every day with kindness.

ANXIETY

20

OVERCOME ANXIETY

"It seems that our life is all past and future, and that the present is nothing more than an infinitesimal hairline which divides them. From this comes the sensation of 'having no time,' of a world that hurries by so rapidly that it is gone before we can enjoy it. But through awakening to the instant, one sees that the reverse is true. It is rather the past and future which are the fleeting illusions, and the present which is eternally real." [53]

– ALAN W. WATTS

Everybody worries about the future to some extent. But in some cases, that worry can turn into anxiety. Approximately 25 to 35 percent of the population suffers from an anxiety disorder.[54]

Have you ever met people who seemed to be blessed with good luck? Even when things don't go their way, they don't seem to worry about it. You can be more like that if you change your thinking and learn how to relax. In this chapter you will learn the causes of anxiety, and techniques for overcoming it.

Ask your doctor or therapist if mind-body relaxation and cognitive therapy are right for you. The techniques in this chapter can complement the work you do with your doctor or therapist, but they should be used in combination with professional guidance.

What Does Anxiety Feel Like?

These are the common symptoms of anxiety.

- Difficulty swallowing, tightness in your throat
- Tightness in your chest, difficulty breathing, or shortness of breath
- Tremors, shakes
- Muscle tension, twitches
- Excessive sweating
- Racing heart, palpitations, arrhythmias, skipped beats
- Dizziness, lightheadedness
- Flushed face, flushed skin
- Numbness, tingling
- Nausea, diarrhea
- Difficulty thinking, speaking, forming thoughts, or following conversations
- Feeling like you are going to faint or pass out

Some medical diseases can also produce these symptoms. I won't list them, because they are less common than anxiety. But if you have any of these symptoms, you should consult your physician.

What causes anxiety symptoms? When you are anxious, your body goes into fight-or-flight mode and releases adrenaline. Adrenaline makes your heart pump faster so that you're ready to fight or run, which makes you prone to skipped beats and arrhythmias. You begin to sweat so that you will be cool if you run. You automatically start taking bigger breaths so that you can take in more oxygen. But that kind of breathing can make you feel as if you're being smothered.

Blood is drained away from the nonessential organs, including your gastrointestinal tract, which makes you feel nauseous. Your brain becomes hyperactive so that you can detect threats quickly, but that makes it hard to think logically. You're more focused on worst-case scenarios.

Depression can cause of anxiety. Approximately 90 percent of people who are depressed also feel anxious. Not everyone who is anxious is depressed, of course. Anxiety can exist on its own without depression. But most people who are depressed are also anxious. (For more on depression, refer to Chapter 23 "Recognize Depression.")

The Two Negative Beliefs That Lead to Anxiety

Anxiety is usually caused by imagined stress instead of real stress. When you see the world in a negative way, you may feel anxious. Two types of negative beliefs lead to most anxiety.

- Thinking that you're not able to face life's challenges because you're flawed or imperfect. Worrying that others will see you as imperfect and judge you.
- Worrying that if something happens, it will be the worst-case scenario. Thinking that if something good happens, you will have to pay for it with something bad.

How High Expectations or Excessive Criticism Can Cause Anxiety

Growing up in a household with overly high standards can make you feel imperfect. You don't need to be criticized to feel flawed. Even the threat of criticism can be enough. Maybe your parents didn't criticize you. But the implication was that people who didn't live up to their high standards weren't good enough.

When you grow up in this kind of environment, you're never quite sure of your own worth. You're not sure if you can live up to those high standards, or if you are flawed and can't succeed. You doubt that you are "good enough." You worry about disappointing yourself or others.

"Look, Dad, I got 95 percent on my exam."

"What happened to the other 5 percent?"

Are you a perfectionist or hard on yourself? Overly high standards lead to all-or-nothing thinking. Anything less than perfect is a failure. The result is that you tend to dwell on your failures and disqualify the positives. You're more worried about avoiding criticism than you are about excelling.

- Did you grow up with someone who was critical of you or others?
- Did you grow up in a household that set very high standards?
- Were you often criticized at school?

How an Unpredictable Childhood Can Cause Anxiety

Growing up in a chaotic or unsafe household makes you expect the worst. This kind of household makes you feel powerless as a child. You're never able to relax because you worry about what will happen next.

To understand this effect, try to imagine living in this household. You don't know one moment to the next what will happen. You spend a great deal of your energy avoiding conflict or chaos. Even when everything is fine, you can't let your guard down because you remember when everybody was screaming at each other. Or worse, you remember when nobody was talking, and nobody would tell you why. You're waiting for the next bad thing to happen. If you grow up in this kind of environment for the first 15 years of your life, you're going to be pretty anxious.

- Did you grow up in a household that was unsafe or unpredictable?
- Was your extended family chaotic or embarrassing?
- Were you bullied as a child?

Thought Record: Social Anxiety

1. The situation.
   Getting ready for a social event.

2. Initial thought.
    I don't fit in at social events. I'm worried that I'll make a fool of myself, or that people won't like me.
3. Negative thinking.
    This is negative self-labeling and all-or-nothing thinking.
4. Source of negative belief.
    I started to think this way in high school, when there was peer pressure.
5. Challenge your thinking.
    I am not the same person I was back in high school. When I show interest in other people, I generally do well in social situations. I feel more comfortable when I'm not trying to impress other people. Many people are just as uncomfortable as I am at these events.
6. Consider the consequences.
    If I continue to avoid these situations, I'll be trapped by my anxiety. I will lose my freedom and become isolated.
7. Alternative thinking.
    I'm sure some people will like something I say if I am sincere. I shouldn't put so much pressure on myself. I don't have to be liked by everyone. Most people aren't.
8. Positive belief and affirmation.
    I have something worthwhile to say. I am likeable.
9. Action plan.
    I'm not going to put pressure on myself. I'm going to be positive and nice to other people, and not expect too much. I will take small steps so that I won't get stuck in all-or-nothing thinking.
10. Improvement. Do you feel slightly better or more optimistic?

Thought Record: Catastrophizing

1. The situation.
    You avoid a necessary conversation with someone because you're afraid they will give you bad news, or you'll have an argument.
2. Initial thought.

I expect the worst to happen. If something good happens, I'll have to pay for it with something bad.

3. Negative thinking.
   This is catastrophizing.
4. Source of negative belief.
   Sometimes I feel like a kid, listening to my parents argue and wondering what will happen. I felt like my whole life fell apart when my parents divorced.
5. Challenge your thinking.
   I know from past experience that the worst rarely happens. Many of the things I worry about are beyond my control. If I look at the big picture, I realize that I'm being overly cautious.
6. Consider the consequences.
   I will be exhausted from all this worrying. Worrying about things I can't control is a waste of my time and energy. I will alienate the people around me by being anxious. I won't enjoy my life.
7. Alternative thinking.
   I know from similar situations that if I do my best and don't get excited I can handle this. I can ask other people how they dealt with this and what their experiences have been to get some perspective.
8. Positive belief and affirmation.
   This may be scary, but I can tolerate a little anxiety. I know it will pass.
9. Action plan.
   If I really need to, I will schedule "worry time." Right now, I'm going to relax for 40 minutes and see how I feel.

The Consequences of Chronic Anxiety

Your body is not meant to be in constant overdrive. The thing about chronic anxiety is that you accept it as the new norm, meanwhile it's still causing emotional wear and tear on your body.

Chronic anxiety depletes neurotransmitters such as dopamine and serotonin, and leaves you mentally and emotionally exhausted.

The physical consequences of chronic anxiety were covered in Chapter 18 "Improve Your Health." Here are some of the emotional consequences:

- Poor concentration
- Irritability
- Exhaustion
- Loss of enjoyment
- Difficulty falling asleep or staying asleep
- Feeling hopeless or pessimistic
- Depression
- Feeling overwhelmed or unable to cope

How Anxiety Affects Your Relationships

When you feel flawed or imperfect, you don't let people close to you. If people get too close they might discover that you're imperfect. They might not like you. Therefore you tend to keep them at a distance.

If you grow up with overly high standards, you may have a high need for approval. You want to forget the past, therefore you look for people who give you approval. You may be overly eager to please. You may have a hard time saying no, or setting healthy boundaries. You'll try to do things for other people even if it means sacrificing what you want. If someone is angry, your first reaction is to think that it's your fault.

If you feel flawed, you may search for unconditional love. The fantasy of unconditional love is that you won't be criticized again, and you'll be able to relax. But that puts unrealistic pressure for your happiness on someone else. As Joseph Campbell said, "Even God doesn't have unconditional love. He throws people into hell."[55]

Instead of expecting unconditional love from others, give yourself unconditional love. Accept yourself for who you are. Acknowledge that you don't have to be perfect. Recognize that your overly high standards are hurting you.

When you expect the worst to happen, you don't allow yourself to feel good. You tend to hold back in life and in relationships. No matter how good things are, you don't allow yourself to be vulnerable, therefore you don't open up in relationships.

Mind-Body Relaxation for Anxiety

Mind-body relaxation helps reduce your anxiety in at least three ways. You recognize how you make yourself anxious. You practice letting go of anxiety. You practice how it feels to be free of anxiety so that you can incorporate that feeling into your life.

If you grew up in a household where you worried about being imperfect or felt powerless, you learned to focus on other people, what they think, and how they can affect your future. In other words, you learned not to live in the moment and not to be in your own skin. Mind-body relaxation helps you overcome anxiety by giving you the chance to practice living in your own skin and being in the moment.

Identify how you make yourself anxious. During a relaxation session, you hear how you talk to yourself. "I expect something bad to happen. I feel flawed or imperfect. I worry that people will judge me." The thoughts that distract you when you try to relax are the thoughts that make you anxious during the day.

You let go of anxiety at the physical level. You can't stop feeling anxious by just thinking you should relax. You let go of your anxiety by turning your focus inward and becoming centered. This releases you from the grip of anxiety.

A mind-body relaxation session helps you practice a healthier way of living. It provides you with a safe environment where you can try letting go of your anxiety and being in the moment. You see what it's like to be free, and that practice gives you the courage to try it in the rest of your life.

The Medical Evidence

Mind-body relaxation reduces anxiety and panic attacks. A study at the University of Massachusetts followed 22 patients who suffered from generalized anxiety or panic disorder. Each patient was taught how to relax. After six weeks, 20 of the 22 participants said they felt significantly more relaxed. The benefits were also long lasting. Three months later, those who continued to practice relaxation reported feeling more relaxed and happy.[56]

Seize the Day

"I went to the woods because I wished to live deliberately ... and see if I could not learn what it had to teach, and not, when I came to die, discover that I had not lived." [57] – HENRY DAVID THOREAU

Seize the day by living in the day, instead of reliving yesterday. Seize the day by letting go of your anxieties and fears so that you are free to seize it.

Most people remember to seize the day only after they've suffered a tragedy or loss. That's when they remember to tell their loved ones how much they love them, and to let go of past resentments. But too often, they forget those lessons until the next tragedy comes along. The idea that life is best lived in the moment is surely one of the most frequently forgotten and rediscovered ideas in history.

The ability to enjoy the moment is the hallmark of a happy life. When people dream of what they'll do when they retire, they dream of living in the moment. They dream of doing the things they want to do and not being in a rush. Then they forget to enjoy the rest of that day, as if living in the moment is a luxury they can postpone.

When you're in the moment, life is sweet. When you're not in the moment, even the most perfect day is hard to enjoy. In the moment is the only place you can feel content and happy. It's where you were meant to live.

Tom is a high-ranking military officer who has sacrificed his personal life for his career. When I saw Tom, he was wondering if it was all worth it. He told me about all the places he'd been, and all the things he had done. I told him that I was impressed with his accomplishments. There was a long silence, and Tom looked away. I looked away too, feeling awkward about intruding on his personal moment.

When I looked back, tears were streaming down his face. When he was able to talk again, he said that he was thinking about all the times he had missed with his family: birthdays, anniversaries, and special events. Even when he was present, he wasn't really there.

He was always anxious to get on to the next thing. But now that he had achieved everything he wanted, he wondered if it had been worth it. He told me how his drinking had escalated to help him deal with his regrets. He wondered if he should have slowed down and enjoyed the small things.

This man with a granite jaw, whom other men would follow into fire, was crying over the simple moments he had missed with his family. He had been so driven to achieve the superficial things that he forgot to pay attention to what really mattered.

Key Points

- There are two basic causes of anxiety: thinking that you're flawed and that you cannot cope, or expecting the worst to happen.
- Growing up with overly high standards can make you feel imperfect and flawed.
- Growing up in a chaotic or unsafe household can make you think that the worst will happen.
- Mind-body relaxation helps you practice letting go of anxiety and living in the moment, which is the only place you can feel content and happy.

21

PANIC ATTACKS

A panic attack is a sudden and intense feeling of fear that usually hits without warning. The effect is so powerful that it can make grown men and women quake with terror. The first panic attack is often the most frightening because you don't know what's happening.

Some people describe panic attacks as a sense of impending doom, or a feeling that they're about to lose control of their minds. In this chapter you'll learn the symptoms and causes of panic attacks, and how to break their hold. Before reading this chapter, please read Chapter 20 on anxiety to learn the necessary background.

The Symptoms of Panic Attacks

A panic attack can include any of the following symptoms:

- Overwhelming fear
- Sense of impending doom
- Tightness in the chest, difficulty breathing, shortness of breath
- Difficulty swallowing, tightness in the throat
- Racing heart, heart palpitations, skipped beats
- Tremors, shakes
- Sweating
- Feeling like you're going to pass out
- Feeling detached or unreal

- Feeling like you're losing control or going crazy
- A fear of dying

The Cause of Panic Attacks

A panic attack – also called an anxiety attack – is a volcano of tension that has built pressure over time, and suddenly erupts. It is preceded by a long buildup phase, when you're under stress without any escape, until eventually you become a wound-up spring, and almost anything can set you off.

The most important thing about a panic attack is the long buildup phase. People sometimes try to identify the trigger of a panic attack, but the triggering event can be almost anything. Once an attack is triggered, your body releases a surge of adrenaline that produces the symptoms of panic.

The buildup phase is the part you should focus on. If you've had a panic attack, think back to the six to twelve months preceding it. Were you under high stress during that time? Did you do anything to relieve your tension?

Once you've had one panic attack, you're more likely to have another. Panic attacks are so frightening that the fear of having another can become a stress in itself that can trigger more.

This is a case that illustrates many of the points of panic attacks. Emily is a teacher who is well liked by her students and peers. While flying to a teacher's conference, she experienced her first panic attack. By the time I saw Emily, she had had more panic attacks and was concerned why they were happening. We began by looking at the first one. Emily reassured me there was nothing stressful about the conference. I asked her to describe her life before the event.

She told me that she and her husband spent every second weekend visiting her aging parents. Her father drank a little too much and was suffering from early Alzheimer's. Emily's brother suffered from depression and had lost four jobs. He sometimes relied on her for money. Emily was a perfectionist who wanted to get the most out of the conference so that she could take the information back to her peers and students.

I suggested that Emily was in survival mode. This was partly due to family circumstances beyond her control, and partly due to her perfectionism. As with all panic attacks, Emily's first one didn't occur out of the blue. She had been under chronic stress for some time. Finally, the stress of flying to the conference, being away from home, and trying to do a perfect job pushed Emily over the edge. Once she had one attack, she was prone to more.

I introduced Emily to mind-body relaxation and cognitive therapy. Within six months she felt she had regained control of her life. What was especially rewarding was that Emily decided to use her new confidence and go to teach in Africa. This had always been her dream, but the panic attacks had prevented her from travelling. After learning how to relax, Emily decided to pursue her dream. As a doctor, I can't think of a greater reward.

How to Prevent Panic Attacks

It's hard to prevent a panic attack just before it's about to happen. The best you can do at that point is manage it by using the techniques I'll discuss in the next section. True prevention involves reducing your tension and changing your thinking during the buildup phase.

Prevention involves cognitive therapy and mind-body relaxation. The goal is to let go of your worries and layers of tension so that you're less like a wound-up spring. It will also help you let go of what you can't control and focus on what you can control.

Write a thorough record about how you contribute to your anxiety and tension. Practice mind-body relaxation every day, and you will see the effect it has on your state of mind.

How to Break the Hold of a Panic Attack

The trick to breaking a panic attack is to get out of your head and into your body. Panic attacks start in your mind and grow in your mind. An attack grows only if you give it room to grow. Therefore the way to break a panic attack is to become grounded in the present. Focus on being grounded and centered, so that you can turn your thoughts away from your panic.

When you have a panic attack, your tendency is to try to mentally run away and hide. You want to run from the feelings, which makes sense when you're confronted with a physical threat. But when you try to hide from your anxiety, you disconnect from the present, which only makes it worse.

This is a technique that works for both panic attacks and post-traumatic stress disorder. (I will discuss post-traumatic stress disorder in Chapter 22.)

- **Lie down in a straight and balanced position.** Your tendency will be to curl up. But try straightening your body so that you don't lock up physical tension.
- **Begin to repeat something to yourself.** Say, "Let go. Let go. Let go." Say it as quickly and loudly as you need to stay focused. Scream it in your mind if you have to, so that you can drown out the noise of your panic.
- **Feel at least five places where your skin touches the ground.** For example, scan your toes, soles, heels, hips, seat, and back. *Feel* your skin touching the ground – don't try to visualize it.
- **Expect to be distracted often.** Your mind will race and dwell on the panic, but don't give up. Keep scanning your body and saying "Let go. Let go. Let go."
- **Scan each area for several breaths before moving on to the next area.** Feel every detail where your skin touches the ground. Your tendency will be to be in a rush. But that will keep you from being in the moment.
- Once you have felt five places, go back and feel at least four places where your skin touches the ground. Then feel three places, then two, and finally one place where you touch the ground.

One of the fears of a panic attack is that it will never end. But an attack is usually short-lived. If you can get through the next 30 minutes, it will usually start to diminish. Knowing that can be a powerful ally.

Key Points

- The buildup to panic attacks occurs when you are under prolonged stress with no escape.
- Once the pressure has built up, a panic attack can be triggered by almost anything.
- Prevention of panic attacks occurs during the buildup phase.
- Mind-body relaxation and cognitive therapy help prevent layers of tension from building.

22

POST-TRAUMATIC STRESS DISORDER

Post-traumatic stress disorder (PTSD) can occur when a person is exposed to severe trauma such as violence or abuse that they are powerless to stop. Some survivors of trauma mentally shut down to avoid feeling any emotions. In a sense, this is a short-term coping strategy that allows the survivor to function. But over the long run, avoiding emotions becomes an obstacle to healthy functioning.

If the survivor doesn't learn coping skills for dealing with their emotions and pain, their post-traumatic stress reaction can turn into a disorder. The suppressed emotions have to come out somehow, and they often come out in the form of anxiety, depression, nightmares, and rage.

The chances of developing PTSD vary greatly, depending on the person and the nature of the trauma. Approximately 9 percent of people exposed to significant trauma in an urban setting develop post-traumatic stress disorder.[58] On the other hand, approximately 20 to 45 percent of combat veterans experience PTSD at some point after war or peacekeeping operations.[59,60]

Please read the previous two chapters on anxiety and panic attacks to learn the necessary background before reading this chapter. *Ask your doctor or therapist if mind-body relaxation and cognitive therapy are right for you.* The techniques in this chapter can complement the work you do with your doctor or therapist, but they should be used in combination with professional guidance.

The Symptoms of PTSD

Do not attempt to diagnose yourself. *If you feel you have some of the following symptoms, you should speak to your doctor or a specialist about PTSD.* Making the diagnosis of PTSD can be subtle and can trigger memories that you may not be able to handle on your own. The main symptoms of post-traumatic stress disorder are the following:

- **Reliving the trauma.** Do you frequently re-experience the trauma in your dreams or flashbacks? Do you act or feel as if you're caught in the traumatic event again? Do you feel intense anxiety when you see or hear people or places that symbolize the trauma?
- **Avoiding triggers.** Do you work hard to avoid people, places, thoughts, feelings, conversations, or anything that can trigger memories of the trauma? Do you have difficulty remembering some important aspect of the trauma?
- **Feeling on guard.** Do you feel constantly on guard? Do you have difficulty falling or staying asleep? Do you have difficulty concentrating? Are you irritable or hypervigilant? Do you startle easily?
- **Feeling detached.** Do you feel detached, numb, or estranged from others? Do you enjoy things less than you did before? Is your range of emotions flatter than before?
- **Diminished sense of the future.** Are you less interested in the future than before? Do you think less about the future, or do you feel more hopeless about the future?

Things You Can Do

"The best way to get rid of your feelings is to feel them."[61] Seek professional help. Find a qualified professional or treatment program with experience in PTSD, and begin to deal with your PTSD.

Take care of yourself. Get enough rest, eat well, exercise, and take time to relax.

Don't self-medicate. Drugs and alcohol temporarily numb your feelings, but they're not healthy coping skills. Drugs and alcohol prevent you from doing the work you need to do to overcome your symptoms. They are also brain depressants, which lead to more problems down the road.

Talk to people. You don't have to talk about your trauma if you don't want to. Just reach out and spend time with your friends and family. Make it clear that you want to keep it light, and you'll talk about deeper issues when you're ready. Connecting with people is healing.

Trust your body. It will tell you how fast or slow you should go in the work you need to do. One of the common fears is that you will open the floodgates and be overwhelmed by your emotions. But your body won't give you more than you can handle generally speaking.

Join a support group. Ask your health care professional about PTSD groups. Look them up in your local phone book, or contact your community social services. A support group will help you feel that you're not alone. You will also learn tips about how other people have dealt with this.

Dealing with Flashbacks

During a flashback, you dissociate from the present and re-experience your trauma. The short-term treatment of flashbacks is the same as that used for breaking panic attacks.

The trick is to get out of your head and into your body. Don't try to escape the scariness of a flashback by withdrawing into your mind. Instead focus on feeling your body. Connect with the present. For a detailed description of how to break flashbacks and panic attacks, please refer to Chapter 21 "Panic Attacks."

Mind-Body Relaxation and Treating PTSD

There are two parts to the treatment of PTSD. The short-term treatment focuses on dealing with flashbacks. The long-term treatment focuses on letting go of your fear and anger so that you can become whole again.

The irony is that as long as you try to avoid the past, it will continue to haunt you. Long-term recovery involves letting go of the past gradually by using the techniques of mind-body relaxation among other things. It involves an overall treatment plan that should include self-care, professional therapy, and support groups.

The main emotions you try to avoid in PTSD are fear and anger. Because you try to avoid them, they come out in powerful bursts. Therefore the long-term treatment involves letting go of your emotions in a safe and controlled way. Peel away your layers one at a time so that they won't come out in bursts. The first step of healing is letting go.

Mind-body relaxation helps you relax and feel safe so that you can let go of your tension. When you try to relax, you will periodically be distracted by tension related to your trauma. When that happens, stop and remind yourself that you're in a safe place.

Separate your tension from everything else you're feeling by naming it. No matter how tempted you are to analyze the past, this is not the time. You are learning how to let go of the past. Do not try to relax your mind. Focus on feeling your skin touch the ground.

Build up to one to two-hour relaxation sessions. Start slowly with a 10-minute relaxation session daily, and add 10 minutes every week. It can take a few months to feel comfortable with longer relaxation sessions. But it takes one to two hours to let go of your deeper layers of fear and anger. That's a long time. But you are trying to regain your life.

You will probably be more anxious in the beginning because you're reluctant to give up control. But relaxation isn't about giving up control. It is about regaining control by letting go of the tension that has been running your life. Although most people prefer to relax with their eyes closed, you may want to keep your eyes open in the beginning.

Accumulated Traumatic Stress Disorder

It's been my experience that some people develop post-traumatic stress disorder, not after one overwhelming trauma, but after many accumulated smaller traumas. If you don't know how to let go of stress, many repeated traumas can have the same effect as one major trauma. This is supported by the fact that not everyone who is exposed to major trauma develops post-traumatic stress disorder.

Adults who develop post-traumatic stress disorder are often the ones who have had painful or traumatic childhoods. In their cases, the final trauma is just the top of many accumulated layers. Past traumas become interconnected so that one triggers another, and older traumas intensify newer ones.

Therefore, I prefer to think of post-traumatic stress as accumulated traumatic stress disorder. This emphasizes the fact that the treatment involves letting go of layers, not just the most recent trauma. Letting go of the past is what sets you free.

Key Points

- Post-traumatic stress disorder can occur when a person is exposed to severe trauma such as violence or abuse that they are powerless to stop.
- Part of the treatment involves letting go of your fear and anger gradually, in a controlled environment, so that you will feel whole again.
- The normal reaction to trauma is to avoid being in the moment. Recovery from PTSD involves relearning how to live in the moment.
- If you don't know how to let go of tension, many repeated traumas can have the same effect as one big trauma.

DEPRESSION

23

HOW TO RECOGNIZE DEPRESSION

"I have studiously tried to avoid ever using the word 'madness to describe my condition. Now and again, the word slips out, but I hate it. 'Madness' is too glamorous a term…. That word is too exciting, too literary, too interesting in its connotations, to convey the boredom, the slowness, the dreariness, the dampness of depression." [62]
– Elizabeth Wurtzel

Depression is an ancient disease that has affected millions of people. As far back as the 4th century BCE, Hippocrates described the symptoms of depression, calling it "melancholia." It has tormented the likes of Winston Churchill, Ernest Hemingway, Abraham Lincoln, and Mark Twain.

Approximately 15 to 20 percent of the population will have at least one episode of depression in their lifetime.[63,64] In North America, the overall burden of depression is greater than that of any other disease. By 2030, it is projected that the disease burden of depression worldwide will be second only to HIV.[65] In this chapter, I will describe the symptoms of depression, and in following chapters you will learn the causes and treatment of depression.

Depression Test

Answer yes or no to the following 10 questions. Most have more than one part because everyone feels depression differently. You need to answer yes to only one part per question in order for that question to count.

1. **Depressed mood.** Do you feel sad, down, or depressed most of the time? Do you feel that all the color has been drained out of your life? Do you cry more easily than usual? Do you have crying spells for no apparent reason?

2. **Loss of interest.** Have you lost interest in things that used to give you enjoyment, or in the activities of your daily life? Have you become more socially withdrawn or isolated?

3. **Low energy.** Do you feel more fatigued or sluggish? Is your energy lower? Is it hard to get going in the morning? Is your libido suddenly reduced, or do you have less interest in sex?

4. **Anxiety. Are you more anxious, worried, fearful, or irritable?**

5. **Lower self-confidence.** Has your self-confidence or self-esteem declined? Do you feel more hopeless or pessimistic than usual? Do you feel more guilty or worthless?

6. **Poor concentration.** Is it hard for you to think, concentrate, or make decisions? Do you find it hard to concentrate on things outside of work? Do you find it harder to read articles, or to absorb what you read?

7. **Sleep changes.** Do you have difficulty falling asleep or staying asleep? Do you feel that you're not refreshed in the morning? On the weekends, do you feel like you could sleep all day and that you don't want to get out of bed?

8. **Appetite or weight change.** Is your appetite either significantly lower or higher than a year ago? Have you unintentionally lost or gained weight? Do you eat only because you have to eat, but find little pleasure in food? Are you doing more emotional eating?

9. **Slow moving or restless.** Are you moving more slowly lately? Is your speech slower? Do you feel like you're shuffling when you walk? Are you more restless or fidgety? Do you wring your hands more than usual?

10. **Thoughts of death.** Do you have recurrent thoughts of death or suicide (not just a fear of dying)? Do you think it would be easier if you just didn't wake up in the morning? Do you think it would be easier if you developed a serious illness? Do you wonder if anyone will miss you when you're gone? Do you think you would be better off dead, or that your family would be better off if you were gone? Do you imagine ways of hurting yourself?

If you answered yes to at least five of these questions, you meet the medical criteria for depression.[66] The most common symptoms are low energy, lack of enjoyment, and high anxiety.

There is no simple blood test for depression. The diagnosis of depression is based on history. The changes that occur with depression go on inside the brain. But they are hard to detect because they occur behind the blood-brain barrier that separates the brain from the blood of the rest of the body. Laboratory tests can determine if there are any other medical causes for depression, such as thyroid disease or diabetes.

How Depression Feels

The best one line description of depression is that it feels like lack of vitality. You don't have to feel sad to be depressed. This is why some people don't seek help for depression. They think they're not depressed because they're not sad. But depression can manifest itself in many ways.

Depression often feels like anxiety. Approximately 90 percent of people who are depressed also feel anxious.[67] Anxiety is such a common symptom that some doctors feel if a patient suffers from anxiety, the first explanation that should be considered is depression.

Patients who are anxious find it difficult to believe that they're depressed. They think their anxiety is making them depressed, but usually it's the other way around. There are other causes of anxiety. But if you are depressed, you will usually feel anxious. (Anxiety is not one of the standard criteria used by the American Psychiatric Association for the diagnosis of depression.)

Depression sometimes feels like irritability. It's been my experience that patients who suffer from depression also feel irritable and intolerant. In fact, when people begin to pull out of depression, they often say they begin to feel more tolerant towards family and friends.

It's only people who haven't suffered from depression who think it isn't real. They underestimate how painful depression can be. They are full of well-meaning advice that isn't always helpful. "Buck up! Pull up your socks!" If you've suffered from depression, you know it's not that simple.

Thoughts of Hurting Yourself

Thoughts of hurting yourself are a frightening but common aspect of depression. Therefore it's important to discuss them openly. Most people who are depressed will have at least some thoughts of dying or hurting themselves.

There is a big difference between having suicidal thoughts and acting on them. *If you have thoughts of hurting yourself, you should immediately discuss them with your health professional.*

There is a difference between active and passive thoughts of hurting yourself. With passive thoughts, you think that it would be easier if you weren't alive. You would prefer to fall asleep and not wake up. But you don't want to hurt yourself. With active suicidal thoughts, you think about hurting yourself. Both are serious, but active thoughts of self-harm are obviously more alarming.

Passive thoughts of hurting yourself are usually fleeting. It's easy to chase them away by remembering that you want to get better, that suicide is permanent, and that you would hurt the people left behind.

Please seek help immediately if your thoughts of death or hurting yourself change in character: if they occur more often, if it's harder to chase them away, or if you start to make plans for hurting yourself. Contact your health professional, call a crisis hotline, or go to an emergency room.

Variations of Depression

There are different levels of depression. People usually assume the worst when they hear depression. They worry that they'll become bedridden or suicidal. But that's the most severe level of depression. Most cases are mild; you can still function and go to work – it's just that your energy and sense of enjoyment are low.

Depression doesn't get worse usually. It's reassuring to know that mild depression will remain mild in most cases. The same is true for moderate depression. Although the symptoms may remain the same, the consequence of depression can progress over time if it is untreated.

The way depression is expressed by each individual depends on many factors, including cultural and personal. Some people don't allow themselves to feel sad. Their depression must come out in other ways.

Some people complain of aches and pains when they're depressed. They go from doctor to doctor looking for an explanation to their symptoms, and are disappointed when none is found. These patients find it difficult to believe that they are depressed. They think their lack of vitality is due to their aches and pains, instead of seeing them as symptoms of depression.

Other people become irritable and intolerant when they're depressed. They're preoccupied with what's wrong with the world, and find fault in things around them.

Another variation of depression is called *dysthymia*, which is a less severe but more chronic form of depression in which your mood is persistently low for at least two years. It can have all the same symptoms of depression, with low-grade dullness and apathy.

Key Points

- Depression feels like a lack of vitality. You don't have to feel sad to be depressed.
- The main symptoms of depression are low energy, low sense of enjoyment, and high anxiety.

24

THE CAUSES OF DEPRESSION

Y ou are not helpless against depression. In fact, most causes of depression are within your control. Knowing this gives you hope that you can overcome it. There are three basic causes of depression:

1. A family history of depression.
2. Drug or alcohol abuse.
3. Feeling trapped in your life.

If you improve your coping skills, you can overcome two of the three basic causes of depression.

A Family History of Depression

Genes explain approximately 30 to 40 percent of depression.[68,69] Numerous studies have looked at identical twins to determine the influence of genes in depression. They have concluded that when one twin becomes depressed, the other twin has a 30 to 40 percent chance of becoming depressed. This means that 60 to 70 percent of the time, depression is due to poor coping skills and environmental factors.

A significant family history of depression is defined as any first- or second-degree relative. This includes parents, grandparents, aunts, uncles, or siblings. If anyone within that circle has had depression, you have a higher chance of developing depression.

How does a family history make you predisposed? Your mood is determined by neurotransmitters such as serotonin and dopamine. If you have a family history of depression, this means the brain chemistry you inherited has a hard time producing these neurotransmitters in the right quantities to keep your mood balanced.

If you think about it, it's a miracle that people don't get depressed more often. Your brain has to produce millions of chemicals every day in exactly the right amounts in order to function properly. If it produces these chemicals in slightly reduced amounts, or not at exactly the right time, you will feel depressed.

A family history of depression can be hard to recognize. Most people don't openly admit that they have had depression. Previous generations barely discussed it. You may have to decide if you have a family history of depression more by observing how people behave, than by what they say.

Substance Abuse and Depression

You have no control over your family history, but you can control whether you take depressants. All drugs and alcohol are brain depressants. In moderate amounts, alcohol does not cause depression. But drug or alcohol abuse does cause depression because it depletes your brain of serotonin and dopamine. Brain scans have shown that it can take months for your brain chemistry to return to normal after drug or alcohol abuse.

Alcohol abuse almost doubles the risk of depression.[70] One study looked at 2,945 alcoholics. Fifteen percent were depressed before they began abusing alcohol. That number jumped to 26 percent after they started abusing alcohol. Once they stopped drinking for an extended period, that rate dropped to 15 percent again. In other words, alcohol abuse almost doubles the risk of depression.

Marijuana users are four times more likely to develop depression.[71,72] One study followed a large group of people for 16 years. It proved that those who smoked marijuana were four times more likely to develop depression than non-marijuana users.

Even stimulants such as cocaine, amphetamines, and MDMA (Ecstasy) can cause depression. Initially, they stimulate your brain, temporarily elevating your mood. But over the long run, they deplete your brain of serotonin and dopamine, causing depression.

Dual Diagnosis

Up to 30 percent of addicts suffer from underlying depression.[73,74] The combination of depression and addiction is referred to as a dual diagnosis or concurrent disorder. People who have a dual diagnosis have a common pattern of staying sober for a while and then relapsing.

If an underlying depression is not treated, recovery from substance abuse feels flat and unrewarding. People who don't have a dual diagnosis, generally start to feel better after stopping using. If a depression is untreated, recovery feels so uncomfortable that people often think of returning to their addiction to escape.

Dual diagnosis is hard to diagnose in the first few months of recovery. It's hard to decide if the symptoms of depression are due to an underlying depression or due to the depressant effect of drugs and alcohol. You usually have to remain abstinent for at least three months before a reliable diagnosis of underlying depression can be made. Sometimes it can take as long as six months for your brain chemistry to begin to return to normal. Of course, these are general guidelines.

How Negative Thinking Makes You Feel Trapped

So far you have learned about the first two causes of depression: a family history and substance abuse. But most cases of depression are due to feeling trapped in your life.

If you feel trapped, you will struggle against that feeling until you either escape or become exhausted and depressed. You can be trapped by external factors, such as a job that you don't like or an unhealthy relationship that won't change. But in most cases, people are trapped by internal factors, such as poor self-esteem or negative self-labeling. Here are some examples of how negative thinking can lead to feeling trapped and lead to depression.

Negative self-labeling can lead to depression. If you think that you're flawed or inadequate, you think that you don't have the ability to be happy. Even worse, you think that you don't deserve to be happy. Self-labeling also creates a vicious cycle that makes you feel more trapped. If you behave as if you're flawed, or take on the "poor me" role, people will respond to you that way. They'll be dismissive, and your self-labeling will become self-fulfilling.

Disqualifying the positives makes you feel trapped. When you disqualify the positives, you focus on how you're surrounded by negatives. A good example of this is never being satisfied with what you have. If you're always chasing after more, the underlying feeling is that you want out of your current life. A little of this can be motivating. But too much will mean that you can't see the positives in your life, which will make you feel trapped.

Of course everybody thinks they will stop when they get what they really want. But many people develop a habit of disqualifying what they have and chasing after more. By the time they get what they had initially wanted, they find it hard to break the habit.

Living up to someone else's expectations can cause depression. When you try to live up to someone else's expectations, you're letting somebody else build a box that you agree to live in. You force yourself to live in that box out of a sense of duty or obligation, but you know that you'd be happier doing something else.

The most common example of this is trying to live up to your parents' expectations. I see a lot of people taking their parents' expectations too literally. They think their parents want them to grow up and have a specific job or make a specific amount of money. Most parents just want their children to be happy. For many people, that can be a liberating realization.

People-pleasing can lead to depression. If you're a people-pleaser, you put everybody's happiness before your own. People may admire your selflessness, and in the beginning, you may enjoy that approval. But eventually you feel trapped.

You're trapped by everyone's expectations. If you take time for yourself, you feel selfish. If you try to slow down, you risk disappointing others. What began as a pleasure becomes a burden.

Excessive "should" statements and being judgmental can lead to depression. You should try to be perfect. People should do the best they can. You shouldn't let other people down. If you are good to other people, they should be good to you.

All those "should" statements divide the world into good versus bad. You draw a circle around the few things you like, and put everything else outside the circle. With each new "should" statements and every new judgment, the circle you feel comfortable in grows smaller, and you feel more isolated and trapped.

Being judgmental doesn't always lead to depression. There are many people who are judgmental and angry but not depressed. But being judgmental takes the joy out of life, which is one of the symptoms of depression.

Medical Causes of Depression

Some diseases and medications can lead to depression. Anemia, diabetes, thyroid disease, and heart disease can cause depression. Long-term use of high blood pressure pills, sleeping pills, or birth control pills can also lead to depression. However, all these situations are less common than the three causes of depression mentioned above.

Your doctor may decide to do blood tests to rule out any medical causes for your depression. These may include complete blood count (CBC), fasting blood sugar, thyroid function, routine electrolytes, vitamin B12, folate levels, and liver function tests. Finally, certain medical conditions can sometimes look like depression; the most common of these is bipolar disorder.

The Difference between Sadness and Depression

Sadness is an appropriate reaction to a negative event. The difference between sadness and depression is that sadness isn't burdened with negative thinking. If you lose your job, it's normal to feel sad. But you'll be prone to depression, if you think that losing your job means that you're a failure, or that you'll never be happy again.

The main difference between sadness and depression is feeling trapped. In sadness, you realize that your situation is temporary, and your self-esteem isn't affected. You realize that it's appropriate to feel low, and you have plans to get out. You do things to pick up your spirits. You talk to friends, get a good night's sleep, and do things that you enjoy. You understand your sadness will get better on its own. Depression, on the other hand, does not get better on its own, and may get worse if left untreated.

This is an example of how feeling trapped can lead to depression. It's the story of Dave and Nicole. They have a blended family with four children from their previous marriages. The children were an issue right from the beginning, but no one talked about it. Nicole's oldest son had attention deficit hyperactivity disorder (ADHD). Dave's daughter smoked marijuana.

Dave and Nicole both hoped that these problems would resolve themselves as the children got older. Instead, things got worse. Both parents argued over how to raise the kids. The kids didn't like each other. It was tense.

Then came the final straw. One weekend, Nicole's son got into trouble with the law. Dave was away when it happened, and when he returned, Nicole didn't tell him about the incident. She didn't want to strain an already difficult situation. As time passed, it became even more difficult for her to admit what had happened.

Eventually the stress of everything wore Nicole down. By the time she came to me, she was sobbing as she told her story. She was depressed because she felt caught between her son and Dave.

The first step was to help her out of feeling trapped. Nicole had to tell Dave about the legal problem. Beyond that, Nicole had to change her all-or-nothing thinking. She felt responsible for everything and everyone. She would feel less trapped if she wasn't as much of a caretaker. Only then would she be taking steps to prevent depression from recurring in the future.

Key Points

- The main causes of depression are a family history, substance abuse, and feeling trapped in your life.
- Most people are trapped by their own negative thinking: all-or-nothing thinking, disqualifying the positives, and negative self-labeling.
- People pleasing can lead to depression.
- Sadness is different from depression, in that it is an appropriate reaction to a negative event.

25

THE ROAD TO RECOVERY FROM DEPRESSION

Y ou can overcome depression and improve your life with a few simple techniques. In this chapter, I will explain how cognitive therapy and mind-body relaxation treat and prevent depression.

Cognitive therapy was originally designed to treat depression. Depression is so uncomfortable that it's hard to imagine you might play a role in the way you feel. You need a technique that will help you understand your thinking, so that you can come up with healthier alternatives and change the way you feel.

Ask your doctor or therapist if cognitive therapy and mind-body relaxation are right for you. The techniques in this chapter can complement the work you do with your doctor or therapist, but they should be used in combination with professional guidance.

Below are two examples of negative thinking that can lead to depression and thought records for overcoming them. The goal of the thought records is to help you see that you are not trapped and find better ways of thinking so that you don't feel trapped in the future.

Thought Record: Poor Self-Esteem

1. The situation.

I don't let people get close to me because I worry they'll discover I'm flawed, or they won't like me. I feel ashamed of who I am.

2. Initial thought.

I feel like a failure. I don't think I have anything to offer. I'm not good enough. If people knew the real me they probably wouldn't like me. Sometimes I feel like a fraud.

3. Negative thinking.

This is negative self-labeling and all-or-nothing thinking.

4. Source of negative belief.

I grew up in a very judgmental environment. When I was growing up, I was told that I wouldn't amount to much.

5. Challenge your thinking.

I will check with other people to make sure that I'm seeing the whole picture, and not focusing on my failures. Everybody is imperfect to some degree. I don't think less of other people because of that. I have succeeded in a number of things, and people have praised me for my successes. I do better when I'm focused on what I can control. I have a number of strengths that I have used in the past.

6. Consider the consequences.

I'm being hard on myself. This is damaging my self-esteem. When I'm hard on myself, I am more likely to sabotage myself and more likely to fail.

7. Alternative thinking.

It's unrealistic to expect that I'll be liked all the time. I don't have to be perfect to be liked. I will fail sometimes, but that doesn't mean I will fail all the time. I will let go of the values I learned growing up. I am a different person now. When I'm in the moment, I'm more successful and more comfortable with who I am. I will not disqualify the positives in my life.

8. Positive belief and affirmation.

I will be kind to myself. What I'm doing is enough.

9. Action plan.

I will practice mind-body relaxation regularly so that I will be more comfortable in myself. I'm going to celebrate my victories, and focus on the positives. Mind-body relaxation will also ensure that I'm relaxed and that I don't slip back into old and familiar thinking.

Thought Record: Loss

1. The situation.
   You've suffered a major loss. It could be a job, a relationship, or a death.
2. Initial thought.
   This is devastating. I don't know if I can bounce back. Things may never be the same. I don't think I'll be happy again.
3. Negative thinking.
   This is disqualifying the positives and catastrophizing.
4. Source of negative belief.
   I was taught that life is a struggle and full of disappointment. I would have to say that one of my parents is fairly negative in their outlook.
5. Challenge your thinking.
   This is a major loss, but I haven't lost everything. I'm focusing on this one loss and minimizing the importance of the many positives in my life. I have strengths that I'm overlooking that will help me rebuild.
6. Consider the consequences.
   If I continue to think like this, it will affect my health. It will prevent me from finding new possibilities. My depression may alienate the people in my life.
7. Alternative thinking.
   It's appropriate that I feel sad. I have to go through the stages of grief (denial, anger, bargaining, depression, acceptance). Therefore I shouldn't expect to bounce back from this loss immediately. I shouldn't avoid grieving. But I don't have to get stuck in this stage either. This is just a transition.
   It's probably true that things will never be the same. Change is inevitable. But if I try to resist change, I will be disappointed.

8. Positive belief and affirmation.
   I deserve to be happy. I am open to discovering something new and different after this transition.
9. Action plan.
   I'll make sure I have the necessary personal and professional supports to help me through this transition, so that I can get ready for the next stage of my life. I'll write a gratitude list, and read it every day.

Exercise: 12 Situations That Can Lead to Depression

Here are 12 situations that commonly lead to depression. The basic theme is that you feel trapped. The remedy is to develop alternative thinking and find a way out of feeling trapped. Go through each case and come up with the alternative approach. I'll start you off with the first case.

1. You don't feel appreciated at work or at home. You feel misunderstood.
   The alternative is to communicate with others to make sure that you're not mindreading. Maybe they appreciate you more than you think. Maybe you're stuck in all-or-nothing thinking. You don't have to be appreciated for everything. You are probably appreciated for some of your qualities. But you'll feel stuck if you think you should be appreciated for *all* your qualities. Finally, don't put too much responsibility for your happiness on other people. Understand that you are responsible for your own happiness and self-esteem.
2. You feel that you don't fit in. You feel that you're not needed or that you're not contributing.
3. You feel caught between two sides. If you agree with one person, you'll disappoint the other person. You feel that you're in a no-win situation.

4. You are overly judgmental and resentful. You feel that others disappoint you.
5. You feel ashamed of who you are. You feel that if people really knew you, they wouldn't like you.
6. You hate your job. You hate the way you look. You hate your life.
7. You're not sure that you deserve to be happy, or if you'll ever be happy.
8. You think other people are happier than you. They have something that you're missing.
9. You feel like you never get a break. Bad things happen to you.
10. You feel responsible for some major negative event, and you think you won't be able to live it down.
11. You feel that you're a disappointment to others or yourself. You feel like a failure.
12. You've suffered a major loss, and you wonder if you'll ever be happy again.

Action Comes Before Motivation

When you're depressed, you have less energy to do things. This can lead to a vicious cycle that causes more inactivity and eventually makes it difficult to do almost anything, including basic chores or making decisions.

What causes this cycle? Depression is associated with negative self-labeling. You don't think that you are capable or worthy of success or happiness. Therefore you interpret your reduced energy as proof that you are a failure. The more you believe that you are a failure, the less active you become. Eventually it can be difficult to do almost anything. How can you break this cycle?

Action comes before motivation. This is one of the profound insights of self-help. Your normal tendency is to wait until you find the motivation to do something. You figure that once you're motivated, you'll be more active. But the opposite is true.

Action is the spur to motivation. Once you do something, you'll be motivated to do more. In fact, once you start doing something, you will often be motivated to do more than you expected. Do something small, and you will gain the motivation to do something bigger later. Don't wait for motivation to strike. Create your own motivation.

Decide *what* you will do, not *how much* you will accomplish.[75] This is the key to creating motivation. Anything you do, no matter how small it might be, is a good beginning. If you prejudge how much you should accomplish, you're sabotaging your recovery with all-or-nothing thinking. Focus instead on what you will accomplish.

Start slowly. Do something new today. Do something else tomorrow. Always keep it small. In fact, do less than you think you can do. This helps you break the habit of all-or-nothing thinking. By doing less than you are capable of, you will still make progress, and you will begin to see yourself in a positive way.

With each action, you will start to believe in yourself, and you'll want to do bigger things. But there's no rush. Just do something, no matter how small. This will put you on the road to recovery.

Affirmations That Support Your Recovery

Disqualifying the positives is a common cause of depression. An effective way to break that habit is with a "gratitude list." Don't be quick to dismiss this suggestion.

There are probably a few negatives in your life, and far more positives. But those few negatives have become a sore spot that you can't seem to ignore. Focusing on those negatives and disqualifying the many positives is a habit you have fallen into.

You will have to change that habit if you want to change your life. A gratitude list is a good place to start. Make a list of five to 10 things that you're grateful for, and read the list every day. This is especially helpful after a relaxation session, when you're more receptive to positive ideas. Do it for a month, and you will see the difference in your thinking.

The opposite of disqualifying the positives is not the naive prescription to just think happy thoughts. Acknowledge and celebrate the positives in your life. You'll be amazed at how effective a gratitude list can be in improving your mood.

How Mind-Body Relaxation Treats Depression

In the previous sections you learned how cognitive therapy helps you understand the negative thinking that makes you feel trapped. But sometimes you already know why you feel trapped. Your problem is that you can't let go of the thinking that makes you feel trapped; you can't stop dwelling on the past or the future.

This is where mind-body relaxation comes in. You practice letting go of things that you can't control and living in the moment so that you won't feel trapped.

Suppose you work in an emotionally dysfunctional workplace. This is a classic example of being trapped by external factors. Yet even here, mind-body relaxation can help.

If you don't know how to relax, you'll go home at night and dwell on what happened during the day. You'll replay the events from the day and fantasize about how to get even. In other words, you will spend precious energy focused on the negatives, instead of looking for a way out. A better strategy is to go home and spend 20 minutes relaxing so that you'll be mentally fresh and more able to look for better alternatives.

The next day, when your frustration builds and you start to think that you're trapped, it will be easier to let it go because you practiced letting it go during your relaxation session.

Mind-Body Relaxation Prevents Depression

Mind-body relaxation prevents depression in a few ways. First, it builds your self-esteem so that you can ignore the negative messages from the past that lead to negative self-labeling. You practice letting go of the fears that developed due to destructive criticism.

Second, it prevents new fears and resentments from building and turning into major obstacles. Finally, mind-body relaxation helps you practice enjoying the moment, which restores your optimism. You practice it so that you can incorporate it into your life.

Depression is so painful that after one episode, you worry you will have another. This worry can become another way you feel trapped. You spend energy worrying about what has happened, instead of being in the present. Mind-body relaxation helps you let go of the past, which reduces the risk of your depression recurring.

The Medical Evidence

Mind-body relaxation reduces the risk of a recurrence of depression by up to 50 percent. One study looked at 55 patients who had recently recovered from depression. They were randomly divided into two groups. Both groups received regular medical follow-up, while one group was also taught mind-body relaxation. Both groups were followed for 60 weeks.

During that time, 78 percent of the non-relaxation group suffered another episode of depression, while only 36 percent of the relaxation group had another depression.[76] The simple act of relaxation can reduce the risk of a recurrence of depression by half.

Antidepressants

It has been proven that the most effective treatment of depression is a combination of psychotherapy and antidepressants.[77] Antidepressants treat the symptoms of depression, while psychotherapy improves your coping skills and reduces the risk of future depression.

Antidepressants help jump-start your recovery. Over the long run, improving your coping skill is the most important way to treat and prevent depression. The problem is that when you're depressed, you can't do the things you're supposed to do. Antidepressants improve your energy, so that you can do the things you must do to pull yourself out of depression.

There are many antidepressants to choose from. Research has shown that no one is better than any other. However, not every antidepressant works for every person. Trial and error is usually involved in finding the right one.

If you are interested in trying antidepressants, discuss them with your doctor. I will discuss only one antidepressant in this book. It is effective, inexpensive, and available over the counter in North America. (It is available only by prescription in parts of Europe.)

St. John's wort is as effective as prescribed antidepressants for the treatment of *mild* depression.[78] This has been proven in numerous studies with thousands of patients. It has also been confirmed in a meta-analysis that looked at the combined results of 37 published trials. The study concluded that St. John's wort is as effective as most antidepressants and has fewer side effects.

Further studies have shown that St. John's wort works in much the same way as prescribed antidepressants. It boosts the uptake of serotonin and dopamine, increasing these neurotransmitters in the brain.

Please remember that this is general medical information, and you should consult with your doctor when making decisions about your health.

Employee Burnout

Burnout is just another word for depression. Employees who are burned out feel exhausted, trapped, joyless, and irritable. They find it difficult to concentrate or make decisions. In other words, they are depressed. Stress and tension play an important role.

The American Institute of Stress estimates that stress and tension cost American businesses $300 billion a year.[79] That cost includes increased health claims, accidents, absenteeism, employee turnover, and reduced productivity.

In the current workplace, people feel they are being squeezed from all sides. They're being asked to do more with less, and they have less time at home. Work-life balance is out of kilter.

I have treated many people for burnout, and the common theme is that they don't know how to relax, and they push themselves to the point of exhaustion. Once people crash, they can take a long time to recover.

Dennis was the sales director at a dysfunctional company, who is now on stress leave. He was a dedicated worker who took his work home with him at night. But his vice-president was a micromanager, and he publicly criticized Dennis at every opportunity.

Executives like Dennis are at greater risk of burnout. They are usually caretakers who are responsible for other people. They learn to anticipate and live in the future. As they get better at their jobs, they often get worse at enjoying life. They can forget to turn off their work skills at home.

Dennis had normal blood pressure when he started the job, but after two years it was through the roof. He joked about it to his co-workers, circulating emails about his head exploding. Eventually, the stress, the micromanagement, and the public ridicule took their toll. Dennis hated his job.

Dennis is now on stress leave. His company is paying him to stay at home and do nothing. The company is not getting the benefits of his expertise, and most of the changes he was supposed to implement are on hold. How productive is that? How much responsibility does Dennis's vice-president bear? Should work performance reviews look at how much tension a person generates in their work area?

Tension affects the bottom line. Stress and tension cost American businesses $300 billion a year. That's a lot of tension. Relaxation makes good business sense. The cost of not teaching people how to relax is too high.

Key Points

- Identify the negative thinking that makes you feel trapped and replace it with alternative thinking.
- Mind-body relaxation has been proven to reduce the risk of a recurrence of depression by up to 50 percent.
- Teaching stress management skills makes good business sense. Employee burnout is usually caused by excessive stress.

ADDICTION

26

UNDERSTAND ADDICTION

"Sometimes a person has to go a very long distance out of his way to come back a short distance correctly." [80] – EDWARD ALBEE

A ddiction is any behavior that you have difficulty controlling, and that you continue to do despite negative consequences. The classic addiction is alcoholism. But this definition applies equally well to drug addiction, gambling addiction, eating disorders, and sexual addiction.

Ten percent of any population suffers from drug or alcohol addiction, which makes addiction more common than diabetes. It crosses all socioeconomic boundaries, and causes pain and suffering in everyone it touches.

Ask your doctor or therapist if mind-body relaxation and cognitive therapy are right for you. The techniques in this chapter can complement the work you do with your doctor or therapist, but they should be used in combination with professional guidance.

Addiction Test

Answer yes or no to the following seven questions. Most questions have more than one part. You only need to answer yes to one part for that question to count.

1 **Tolerance.** Has your use of drugs or alcohol increased over time?

2 **Withdrawal.** When you stop using, have you ever experienced physical or emotional withdrawal? Have you had any of the following symptoms: shakes, sweats, nausea, vomiting, irritability, or anxiety?

3 **Difficulty controlling your use.** Do you sometimes use more or for a longer time than you would like? Do you sometimes drink to get drunk? Does one drink lead to more drinks?

4 **Negative consequences.** Have you continued to use even though there have been negative consequences to your relationships, family, job, health, mood, or self-esteem?

5 **Neglecting or postponing activities.** Have you ever put off or reduced household, social, work, or recreational activities because of your use?

6 **Spending significant time or emotional energy.** Have you spent a significant amount of time obtaining, concealing, planning, or recovering from your use? Have you spent a lot of time thinking about using? Have you ever concealed or minimized your use? Have you ever thought of schemes to avoid getting caught?

7 **Desire to cut down.** Have you sometimes thought about cutting down or controlling your use? Have you ever made unsuccessful attempts to cut down or control your use?

If you answered yes to at least three of these questions, you meet the medical criteria of addiction.[81]

It may seem that this is an easy test to fail. If you applied this test to other aspects of your life, you would almost certainly conclude that you're addicted to something. For example, many people watch too much television, or eat too much of their favorite food. But these are so-called soft addictions, and the above test was not designed for them. This test is very reliable when it comes to assessing drug and alcohol addiction.

Understanding the Test

What do these questions say about addiction? Let me explain them in terms of alcohol addiction, but the principles apply to all addictive substances.

1. Tolerance. If your drinking has increased over time, this has put a strain on your body, specifically your liver. Moderate drinkers don't develop tolerance. They may drink slightly more on special occasions, but most of the time they drink roughly the same amount.

2. Withdrawal. Withdrawal does not include hangovers, which even moderate drinkers can get. But shakes and sweats are a sign that your body has been stressed by alcohol. You have to drink a fair bit in order to feel shaky or sweaty the next day.

Emotional withdrawal is just as significant as physical withdrawal. The symptoms of emotional withdrawal include irritability and anxiety, which once again, moderate drinkers do not experience.

3. Difficulty controlling your use. This is the most important criterion of all. It means that alcohol gives you a buzz that you chase after. You may not have difficulty controlling your use every time. But if you sometimes drink more than you would like, this says that your brain is wired differently than a moderate drinker. Your brain feels alcohol differently.

The effect that each person feels when they drink alcohol is mostly determined by genetics. What goes on inside your brain is different from what goes on inside a moderate drinker's brain. This is why you can't understand each other.

A moderate drinker doesn't get the same buzz therefore they don't find it difficult to control their drinking. After a few drinks, they are happy to stop. After a few more, they don't even like the feeling. Meanwhile, you're just getting started.

If you have difficulty controlling your drinking, your drinking has become unpredictable. All the negative consequences you are likely to experience follow from this essential fact.

4. Negative consequences. This means that alcohol causes pain in your life, but you keep drinking because you're chasing the buzz.

Begin by looking at the consequences to your relationships and self-esteem. Don't begin with the consequences to your work because that's usually the last part of your life to suffer.

You are probably careful to avoid affecting work because your employer is the least tolerant person in your life. When alcohol begins to affect your work, you have slipped from being a functioning alcoholic to a non-functioning alcoholic.

5. **Neglecting or postponing activities.** This says that you're willing to trade off part of your life to make more room for drinking. In the beginning, it won't be big things. It's usually little things like household chores. But this is the thin edge of the wedge. If you're willing to trade off small things for drinking now, you may trade off bigger things later. Perhaps you have already experienced this gradual progression.

6. **Spending significant time or emotional energy.** The best example of this is concealing or minimizing your drinking. You know that there's something wrong, but you don't want people to interfere with it.

Often, it's not outright lying. When someone asks you how much you drank, you tell them that you drank less than you really did. Another common example is living a double life to make more room for drinking. Have you ever thought up schemes to avoid getting caught? If so, your alcohol use has begun to take control of your life.

7. **Desire to cut down.** When was the first time that you thought you drink too much? Did you try to cut down, only to have your drinking slowly escalate again? Have you tried to control your drinking, hoping that this time would be different? This is the insanity of addiction: doing the same thing, and expecting a different result.

An alcoholic eventually discovers that it's easier to quit drinking than it is to control their drinking. Controlling your drinking is hard work. Living a sober life is easier, once you realize that alcohol doesn't define you.

There are degrees of addiction. The most extreme case is the non-functioning addict. They have lost their job, and have to use every day. This is the stereotype, but it's rare.

The more common case is the functioning addict. They still have a job, but their life and relationships are starting to suffer. You don't have to suffer major losses to have an addiction. If you wait until you reach that point, it will become harder to rebuild your life.

The consequences of addiction get worse over time. Addiction is a progressive disease. It's never easy to quit. But if you have suffered negative consequences already and don't want them to get worse, there's never a better time to quit than now.

What Addiction Is Not

There are a number of misconceptions about addiction. They all portray the stereotype of addiction, rather than what addiction is really like. Unfortunately, people often refer to these misconceptions as a way of proving that they don't have a problem.

You don't have to use every day. In fact, there is nothing in the definition about how often you use. You may use only once a month. However, if on those occasions, you sometimes have difficulty controlling how much you use, or if your drinking leads to negative consequences, then you have an addiction.

You don't have to crave drugs or alcohol. You may go for a whole month without thinking about using or having cravings. But if you have difficulty moderating your use, you still have an addiction.

You don't have to go through withdrawal. Every person is different when it comes to physical withdrawal. Some people experience significant withdrawal, and others experience very little. There is little correlation between how much physical withdrawal you experience and the extent of your addiction.

You don't have to suffer major losses. If your family members have ever commented on your use, you've already suffered significant losses. In the beginning, it takes all their courage to make the smallest comment about your use. The look of disappointment in their eyes is a loss. Bigger losses are harder to repair. By the time you've suffered major losses, you have a major addiction.

You don't need a fancy definition to tell you if you have an addiction. There is a simple test. If you think you might have a problem, you probably do.

The Causes of Addiction

Addiction is due 50 percent to genes and 50 percent to poor coping skills.[82] This has been proven by a number of studies. Most genetic studies compare the rate of addiction among twins. If one identical twin is addicted to alcohol, it is known that the other twin has approximately a 50 percent chance of being addicted as well. But if a fraternal (non-identical) twin is addicted, the other twin has approximately a 10 percent chance of being addicted. Based on these differences we can conclude that 50 to 60 percent of addiction is due to genetic factors.[83]

A significant family history of addiction is defined as any first- or second-degree relative. This includes parents, grandparents, aunts, uncles, or siblings. If anyone in that circle has had an addiction, you have a higher chance of developing one as well.

Children of addicts are eight times more likely to develop an addiction than the children of non-addicts.[84] One study looked at the first-degree relatives (parents, siblings, or children) of addicts versus non-addicts. The results showed that children who had a parent with a drug or alcohol addiction were eight times more likely to develop an addiction themselves.

If you are predisposed to addiction, this means that your brain is wired differently than that of a non-addict. You get a different buzz from drugs and alcohol.

Repeatedly abusing drugs or alcohol permanently rewires your brain.[85] Even if you have a low genetic predisposition, you can still develop an addiction. If you repeatedly abuse drugs or alcohol because of poor coping skills, you will permanently rewire your brain. Every time you abuse alcohol, you'll strengthen the wiring that gives you an alcohol buzz, and you'll move one step closer to addiction.

Your genes are not your destiny. If you come from a family with a history of addiction, you can avoid developing an addiction by learning good coping skills. Many people have come from addicted families but managed to overcome their family history and live happy lives.

Disease versus Choice

Some people feel that addiction is a choice. They think that since addicts choose to drink, they can choose not to drink. On the other hand, most addicts feel that addiction is a disease. They have difficulty controlling their drinking because their brain is wired differently. It's one of the most contentious issues between addicts and their families.

Addiction is both a disease and a choice. Both statements are correct. Addiction is a disease in that the brain of an addict feels drugs differently than the brain of a non-addict. That buzz is genetically determined and cannot be changed. On the other hand, using drugs or alcohol is a choice, and addicts can choose to stop and change their lives. They can choose to learn new coping skills.

Both statements are correct because they refer to different stages of drinking. Addiction is a choice before you pick up the first drink – but a disease after that.

Are you powerless against your disease? You may have heard the term "powerless" used in 12-step literature. It's a misunderstood point that I want to explain because it prevents people from properly treating their addiction.

You are more powerful than your addiction, in that you can change your life. You are not defined by it. At the same time, there is one part of your addiction that is more powerful than you. You cannot change the wiring of your brain, or the buzz you get from drugs and alcohol. You cannot change your genetic makeup. Sooner or later, one drink will lead to more drinks, even if you learn new coping skills. Therefore, recovery requires total abstinence.

Certain parts of the brain are capable of changing. This is called neuroplasticity, and explains how you can learn new things. However, while you can add memories, you cannot erase them. Once you have experienced the buzz of alcohol, you cannot erase that memory pathway from the pleasure center of your brain.

The question of whether addiction is a disease is one of the most important in recovery. Not understanding it has probably led to more relapses than any other issue. I encourage you to do a thought record on this question every month for the first year, and see how your understanding of addiction grows.

Cross Addiction

If you are addicted to one drug, you can become addicted to another drug. Your addiction can switch from marijuana to alcohol, or from alcohol to cocaine. Cross addiction occurs because all addictions work in the same part of the brain. If your brain is wired for one addiction, you are predisposed to all addictions. If your current drug of choice is taken away, you will probably find a substitute.

Cross addiction is especially prevalent in women who come from alcoholic families. They often develop addictions that go undetected, such as addictions to tranquilizers, pain relievers, or eating disorders.

One drug can make you relapse on another drug. This is one of the consequences of cross addiction. Suppose you're addicted to cocaine. If you want to stop using cocaine, you have to stop using all addictive drugs, including alcohol and marijuana. You may have never had a problem with either of them. But if you continue to use them, even casually, they will eventually lead you back to your drug of choice.

How does cross addiction lead to relapse? First, all addictions work in the same part of the brain. Therefore one drug can trigger urges for another drug. Second, even moderate drinking or marijuana use lowers your inhibitions, which makes it harder for you to make the right choices.

Finally, if you stop using your drug of choice but continue to use alcohol or marijuana, you're saying that you don't want to learn new coping skills. In essence, you're saying that you don't want to change your life. You want to rely on drugs or alcohol to escape, relax, and reward yourself. But if you don't learn new skills, then nothing will have changed. And whatever brought you to your addiction will eventually catch up with you again.

Exercise: 20 False Statements about Addiction

These are common negative thoughts that are obstacles to recovery. None of these statements are true. But negative thinking makes you think they are. I encourage you to do a thought record on each example, and begin to change your thinking about these important topics.

1. I don't have an addiction. I can stop any time I want.
2. Most of my friends would fail this addiction test. We can't all be addicts.
3. What's the harm in using once in a while? It helps me relax at the end of the day.
4. I can't imagine never using again, so I might as well keep using.
5. Maybe I have an addiction. But I need to use drugs or alcohol to deal with my problems. It's easier to feel numb than to deal with my life the way it is.
6. Addiction is fun. It feels good to be bad. My life would be boring without drugs or alcohol. I wouldn't be as interesting or funny or creative, and I wouldn't be as smooth at social events.
7. I haven't hit rock bottom. Maybe I have to keep using before I can find the motivation to quit.
8. I doubt that I can overcome my addiction. There's no point in trying. Maybe it's better that I don't fully commit to recovery. What if I can't succeed?

9. The last relapse was so scary that I don't want to use again. I don't need more help to stay clean and sober.

10. I want to overcome my addiction. But I want to prove to myself that I am strong enough, and that I can beat this thing on my own.

11. I can't quit now. I'm in too deep.

12. I don't think I can cope with my cravings. I don't think I'm strong enough.

13. I don't see relapses coming. I'm fine one moment, and the next moment I'm using.

14. Now that I've relapsed a little, I might as well keep going.

15. I'm so busy that I don't have time to relax or take better care of myself.

16. If I have to change my whole life to overcome my addiction, I don't think I have the energy or the strength.

17. When I'm about to relapse, I don't ask for help because I don't want to be talked out of using.

18. What's wrong with relapsing a few times a year? Maybe I have an addiction. But why not blow off a little steam every now and then? I'm just quitting to make my spouse happy.

19. I have so much fun using with my friends. I can't get rid of them all.

20. Maybe after I have stopped using for a year and I feel stronger, I'll be able to control my use.

Here are some alternative thoughts to get you started. It's never too late to quit. There are always more negative consequences waiting for you if you continue to use.

No relapse is good. But a small relapse has fewer consequences than a big one. Don't turn a little mistake into a big mistake. If you slip, stop and ask for help.

You don't have to change your life all at once. Start with one thing. Start with the easiest thing. Once you start to improve one area of your life, the rest will follow.

Don't think about quitting forever. Even addicts in long-term recovery don't think like that. It's too much to handle. Do your recovery one day at a time. Don't sabotage your recovery by taking big steps. I am struck by how old *and* modern this idea is. Each generation has had to rediscover this truth. A thousand years ago, Chinese philosophers said, "On a long journey take small steps." We now say, "Don't sabotage yourself with all-or-nothing thinking." The principle is the same.

The Opportunity for Change

Your addiction has given you the opportunity to change your life. The fact that you have to change your life is what makes recovery both difficult and rewarding. It's difficult because you have to change your life, and all change is difficult – even good change.

On the other hand, recovery is rewarding because you get the chance to change your life. Most people sleepwalk through life. They don't think about who they are or what they want to be, and then one day they wake up and wonder why they aren't happy.

People in recovery often describe themselves as grateful addicts. You may wonder why someone would be grateful to have an addiction. Because recovery has allowed them to find an inner peace and tranquility that most people crave. Recovery is your opportunity to be happier. You can look back on your addiction as one of the best things that ever happened to you.

Key Points

- Addiction is any behavior that you have difficulty controlling, and that you continue to do despite negative consequences.
- You don't have to use every day, or have cravings to have an addiction.
- Addiction is both a disease and a choice. Addiction is a choice before you pick up the first drink – but it's a disease after that.
- Cross addiction implies that one drug can make you relapse on another drug.
- You are not alone. Many people have overcome their addiction. All of them had moments of despair. All of them doubted their strength. But in the end they succeeded, and are now enjoying a new life. It can be done. You can do it too.

27

THE FIVE RULES OF RECOVERY

"All great truths are simple in the final analysis,
and easily understood; if they are not, they are not great truths." [86]
– Napoleon Hill

Recovery is not easy, but it is simple. It's not due to chance, but governed by a few basic rules. If you follow these five rules, you will do well and enjoy your life. If you don't follow them, you probably won't.

I developed these rules while trying to understand why some people do well in recovery, while others don't. It has become one of my most requested lectures. If you have relapsed in the past, this chapter will help you understand what went wrong, and what you can do differently.

Rule 1: You Must Change Your Life

You don't recover from addiction by just stopping drugs or alcohol. You recover by creating a new life where it is easier to not use. I have worked in addiction medicine for over twenty years, and I believe this is the most important thing that patients and their families need to understand. If you don't create a new life, then all the factors that brought you to your addiction will eventually catch up with you again.

You don't have to change your entire life. There are just a few behaviors that have probably been causing you trouble, and they will continue to get you into trouble until you change them. The more you try to hold onto your old life, the less well you will do in recovery.

The first rule is about creating a secure recovery. If you change your life, then many things will have to fail before you relapse. If you don't change your life, the slightest mistake can lead to problems.

The Neuroscience Behind Rule 1

Recovery is a struggle between your upper and lower brain. The urge to use drugs or alcohol comes from your primitive brain. The desire to stop using and improve your life comes from your upper brain.

Addiction feels like there are two voices inside your head; an angel on one side and a devil on the other. Your primitive brain is screaming for the next hit, while your upper brain is arguing for abstinence and long-term happiness. It's the classic struggle between pleasure and happiness.

The reason you must change your life is because urges from your primitive brain can overpower the logic of your upper brain. The primitive brain has not evolved in a 100 million years, and it is driven by strong emotions such as anger and pleasure. Your upper brain uses logic, which is no match for them.

You have to avoid getting into a power struggle with your primitive brain if you want to have a stable recovery. You can't persuade your primitive brain with logic. It is relentless in its desire to seek pleasure. You can't beat it. Therefore, you have to work around it.

This is why advice like, "Just say no to drugs," is so hard to follow. That kind of advice appeals to the logic of your upper brain. But it doesn't give you a strategy for overcoming the urges from your lower brain.

When you create a new life where it's easier to not use, you are working around your lower brain. Your higher brain creates this life so that your lower brain will not be triggered as much. Part of creating that new life is avoiding high-risk situations.

HALT

High-risk situations can be divided into two types: internal and external. Internal high-risk situations are best described by the acronym HALT:

- Hungry
- Angry
- Lonely
- Tired

How do you feel at the end of the day? You're probably hungry because you haven't eaten well. You're probably angry because you've had a tough day at work. You may feel lonely because you're isolated. You don't have to be physically alone to feel lonely. And you're tired. This explains why your strongest cravings for drugs or alcohol usually occur at the end of the day.

The most common external high-risk situations are people, places, and things:

- People who you used with
- Places where you used, or where you got drugs or alcohol
- Things that remind you of using

How can you avoid high-risk situations? You can't avoid them altogether. But by taking better care of yourself you can avoid some HALT situations. You can avoid being hungry at the end of the day by eating a healthier lunch. You can avoid feeling isolated by joining a 12-step group. You can avoid feeling angry by learning how to relax and let go of resentments quickly. You can avoid being tired by going to bed early.

Make a list of your high-risk situations. Addiction is sneaky. Sometimes you won't see a high-risk situation until you're right in the middle of it. Therefore learn to look out for them. Make a list of your high-risk situations and go over it with someone in recovery to make sure you haven't missed anything. Keep that list with you. One day, it may save your life.

Rule 2: Be Completely Honest

An addiction involves lying. There's no getting around it. You have to lie about getting your drug, using it, and planning your next relapse. Addiction is all about lying. In fact, you're probably so used to lying that you lie even when you don't have to.

But lying comes at a price. You have lied so much that by now you have ended up lying to yourself. You may feel lost or that you don't know who you are. The final victim of your lying is you. When you lie, you can't like yourself or look yourself in the mirror. But you can find yourself again.

Recovery requires complete honesty. You must learn to be 100 percent honest with the people in your life. Who must you be honest with? You need a recovery circle that should include your family, doctor, therapist, 12-step group, and sponsor. If you can't be completely honest with those people, you won't do well in recovery.

Lying leaves the door open for relapse. When you are completely honest, you don't give your addiction room to hide.

Show common sense about disclosing your addiction. You don't have to be completely honest about your recovery with everyone. Not everyone is your best friend, and not everyone will be supportive of your recovery.

But don't feel ashamed to discuss your recovery with the people close to you. You should only feel ashamed if you don't do anything about your addiction, and you ruin your life and the lives of the people who love you.

What does being 100 percent completely honest mean? It means you are completely honest from the present forward. It doesn't mean you have to go back and rehash everything you did in the past. In some cases that can be more harmful than good. But that doesn't let you off the hook about being honest in the future.

One mistake people make is to assume that honesty means being honest about other people. They think they should point out what's "wrong" with other people. But recovery isn't about fixing others. It's about fixing yourself. Stick with your own recovery. Focusing on other people is just a way to deflect attention from yourself.

In the beginning, honesty won't come naturally. You've spent so much time lying that telling the truth, no matter how good it is for you, won't be easy. You will know that you're making progress, when you stop yourself in the middle of a story, and say, "Now that I think of it, it was more like this..."

Rule 3: Ask for Help

Addiction grows by encouraging shame and isolation. Recovery involves reaching out and asking for help from people in recovery.

There are many sources of help in recovery, including doctors, therapists, addiction counselors, and treatment programs. Most of those are easy to understand. I will focus on how 12-step groups can help.

There are few places in the world where you will find more honesty and support than a 12-step group. It's one of the most amazing experiences you can have. Twelve-step groups are an important part of recovery for two reasons. First, they have already helped millions of people. Second, they're free and universally available. Almost every country, city, cruise ship, and small town has a 12-step group.

How Can 12-Step Groups Help?

Twelve-step groups help you decide if you have an addiction. You get to hear other people's stories and see if there are any similarities between theirs and yours.

Twelve-step groups help you overcome your denial by showing you that addiction can affect anyone. Good people with jobs, families, and a sense of humor can have an addiction. You may know this intellectually, but you need to see it to believe it. Everybody likes to think they're special, but addiction is one of those cases when it's comforting to know that you're not alone.

You meet other people who are going through the same thing. The idea behind a 12-step group is that you feel stronger when you are with others who are doing the same thing. If you are like most people, your first instinct will be to deal with your addiction on your own. But that contributes to the isolation and sense of shame of addiction.

Addicts know shame because they often grow up in households that operate on shame and criticism. Using drugs and alcohol feeds that shame, which makes the addict withdraw further and creates more room for the addiction to grow. Reach out and ask for help.

You will see that recovery is possible. Learn how other people have dealt with their addiction. You may worry that your life will be smaller or less interesting without drugs or alcohol. Twelve-step groups give you a chance to meet people whose lives are bigger and more interesting now that they've stopped using.

You learn about other people's recovery techniques. Twelve-step meetings are a resource. You can ask other people how they handled certain situations, and if what you're going through is normal. Some days you'll have an overwhelming urge to use, and it's good to know that other people have gone through the same thing. You can learn what techniques they used to beat it.

You won't be judged. Most addicts have difficulty sharing their emotions because they're afraid they won't be understood. They bottle everything up inside, which makes them want to use even more. The people at a 12-step group won't judge you because they've heard it all before. They've done it all before. They won't think you're crazy. They know what it means to have an addiction.

You're reminded of the consequences of using. I can promise you that this will happen. After you've been clean and sober for six or 12 months (it usually happens around those times), you'll feel stronger than you've felt in years. And that's when the voice of your addiction will tell you that you can control your use now. This time will be different.

At 12-step meetings you will hear from people who relapsed that way. They will tell you that they felt they could control their use. You will be reminded that addiction is a disease. If you had heart disease, you would never think that once you started feeling better, you were no longer at risk, and you could eat anything you wanted. If you had diabetes, you would never think that you could stop taking your insulin once you started feeling better. Twelve-step meetings remind you of this fact.

You have a safe place to go. Twelve-step meetings are a safe harbor where you can go to be out of harm's way. The meetings are usually held in the evening when you probably have your strongest urges for using. If you've had a bad day, you can go to a meeting and spend a couple of hours with like-minded people. By the end of the meeting, you'll almost certainly feel better and more motivated for recovery.

Twelve-step groups are a source of hope, strength, safety, and guidance.

Some Myths about 12-Step Groups

Twelve-step groups do not define you as weak or powerless. They show you that you have the power to regain your life. They do not label you or shame you. They encourage you to let go of shame, by treating addiction like a disease. While your addiction encourages you to withdraw and avoid help, 12-step groups will encourage you to ask for help and change your life.

Finding the Right Group

Every group is different. They each have their own personality and their own mix of people. Some groups you will like, and some you won't. Finding the right group is important because it helps you get the most out of a meeting.

Don't keep going to a group that you don't like just because it's convenient. If you do, you'll eventually convince yourself that you don't need to go to meetings. (The meetings in your area are listed on the Internet. I have included a list of 12-step group websites on www.AddictionsAndRecovery.org.)

There is a simple technique for finding the right group. Go to a meeting, and find someone who you have something in common with. Ask them what other meetings they like. It's a common question, so don't feel embarrassed to ask. Then go to one of those meetings, and do exactly the same thing. Find somebody else, and ask them what other meetings they like. Do that a few times, and you will quickly zero in on meetings that work for you.

Get the Most Out of Your Group

Be active. Recovery doesn't come from just going to meetings. The magic of recovery happens when you participate at meetings, when you share what you're feeling, and when you're honest – uncomfortably honest.

There are two types of 12-step meetings: open (also called speaker meetings), and closed (also called discussion meetings). In speaker meetings, someone stands up and tells their story of addiction and recovery. The beauty of speaker meetings is that you're not expected to say anything. Therefore they're a non-threatening way to get started. The downside is that you don't get to talk or do any work.

Become active by going to discussion meetings. But don't worry. You don't have to say anything if you don't want to in the beginning. You can pass. In fact, it's normal to go a few times and just observe.

Be committed. Join a group and go to it regularly. How often should you go? There is no one answer. Most people like to go to at least two meetings a week in the beginning. Some people like to go every day. Everyone's needs are different. But once a week is probably not enough in the beginning because you will have frequent urges.

Go to meetings on the days that you used. Your body has an internal clock, and if you drank every Friday at 6 o'clock, that's when you'll have your strongest urges to use.

Accept people's offers of help. People will offer to help in many ways. They'll offer to get together and talk about your problems, or they will offer their phone number in case you want to talk any time, day or night. They've been through it before, and they know that recovery is hard work.

In the beginning, you may be overwhelmed by such generosity. But their offers are sincere. They know that by helping you, they're also helping themselves. When they listen to your stories, they are reminded of where they've been and what they need to do to remain clean and sober.

Finding a Sponsor

Get a sponsor and do step work. A sponsor is your own personal coach or teacher to help you through recovery. There are two types of sponsors. A temporary sponsor is a support to help you get started into 12-step groups. They can explain the format of meetings, or suggest a meeting to try. They can also act as an early warning system to help you recognize if you're moving toward relapse. You can have more than one temporary sponsor.

A full sponsor is a teacher to help you go through the 12 steps. A sponsor is someone whom you respect for their recovery and serenity. They don't necessarily have to be your friend. You will find your sponsor by going to many meetings, and hearing people speak and seeing how they behave.

A sponsor should meet a few basic criteria. A sponsor should preferably have at least five years of recovery to have a good perspective. A sponsor should also be someone with whom there is no chance of developing romantic feelings in either direction.

Interview your potential sponsor. The sponsor-sponsee relationship is a close one, and it's important that you find someone who you can work with. I encourage you to interview each other before committing to working together. Begin by asking your potential sponsor an open-ended question. "Tell me what you do with your sponsees?" It's inquiring without putting either of you in an awkward position.

You're looking for someone who has the time to meet at least once a week. You want someone who will give you homework and guidance to help you understand the 12 steps. Beyond that, the rest is a matter of personal preference.

The 12 Steps

I want to make a few comments about the 12 steps. Entire books have been written about them, and there are study guides to help you go through them. Therefore my comments will be brief.

Only the first step is about addiction. The other 11 steps are about understanding yourself and how you got here. I am struck by the similarity between the 12 steps and the steps of a cognitive therapy thought record. They both help you understand the negative thinking that contributed to your addiction. They help you replace your negative thinking with healthier thinking, and incorporate your new thinking into your life.

You don't have to be an addict to benefit from the 12 steps. The world would be a better place if we all followed them. But when a non-addict doesn't follow the principles of the 12 steps, it leads to unhappiness. When addicts don't follow the 12 steps, they end up relapsing in order to escape their unhappiness.

Rule 4: Relax Every Day

Addicts use drugs and alcohol to escape, relax, and reward themselves. Those are the main reasons why addicts use. In other words, they use to deal with tension. Everyone needs to escape, relax, and reward themselves. Those are essential coping skills for a happy life. But addicts don't know how to do those things without using.

If you stop using drugs and alcohol but don't learn how to relax, then all the stresses that brought you to your addiction will still be there. Your fears and resentments will eventually make you feel so uncomfortable that you will relapse just to escape. Tension is the most common cause of relapse.

When you are tense, you will do what is familiar and wrong. It won't take much to push you over the edge. It will be some dumb little thing at the end of a stressful week, and you'll say to yourself, "That's it. I can't take it anymore.

Consider the story of Mike. He has a stressful job and a young family of three children. He loves his family, but sometimes he can't face the idea of going straight home after work. He needs to unwind.

So he buys a bottle of vodka, parks his car a block away, and drinks the whole bottle before facing the rest of his evening. His wife is upset because he arrives home drunk. His children get short-changed because he doesn't spend much time with them. Mike knows all these things. But he keeps relapsing.

What does Mike need to change? He needs healthy alternatives to what he's getting from alcohol. He needs to find better ways, to escape, relax, and reward himself. Mind-body relaxation can be part of that plan.

Mind-Body Relaxation Is Essential to Recovery

Mind-body relaxation is not an optional part of recovery – it is essential. I cannot emphasize this enough. It is probably the most important coping skill in recovery.

I know mind-body relaxation will help. I have treated thousands of patients. Many of them have told me that mind-body relaxation has changed their lives. The only reason people don't relax is because they think they're too busy to relax. It goes something like this: "I know it makes sense, but I've got so many other things I have to do."

Ask yourself how much time you spend on your addiction. If you add up all the hours it takes to get your drug, use it, hide the evidence, and plan your next relapse, relaxing for 20 to 40 minutes a day is a bargain. I promise you will save time, and do better in your recovery.

- Mind-body relaxation improves your self-esteem so that you have less reason to turn to drugs and alcohol.
- It helps you let go of fears, resentments, and emotional pain that contribute to addiction.
- It gives you a healthier way to escape, relax, and reward yourself.
- It is the basis of self-care. You learn to put time aside just for you.
- It reduces the risk of relapse by making it easier to do what's new and right, instead of repeating what's familiar and wrong.

The Medical Evidence

There is overwhelming medical evidence that mind-body relaxation helps recovery. Numerous studies have shown that relaxation reduces the use of alcohol, tobacco, and marijuana.[87]

One study looked at 126 individuals who abused alcohol. After practicing mind-body relaxation for two years, 40 percent reported they had stopped drinking. After three years, 60 percent reported they had stopped using.[88]

Another study reviewed 24 research articles that looked at the benefits of relaxation in recovery. It concluded that mind-body relaxation is effective in preventing and treating substance abuse, and in improving self-esteem.[89]

Research indicates that mind-body relaxation mimics the calming effects of alcohol and tranquilizers. Alcohol and tranquilizers work by stimulating the release of GABA (gamma-aminobutyric acid), the main calming neurotransmitter in the brain. Research indicates that mind-body relaxation also stimulates the release of GABA.[90]

Rule 5: Don't Make Your Own Rules

There are five rules of recovery. The fifth rule may not sound like the others, but it is just as important. It reminds you not to do things your way. You've tried to deal with your addiction your way. It didn't work! Why not try something different?

Don't look for loopholes in recovery. You will know if you're trying to do recovery your way, if you catch yourself looking for loopholes. Recovery requires commitment. Sometimes you will be tested. You have to expect that recovery will sometimes be hard. But it's easier than active addiction.

You'll know that you're looking for loopholes if you focus on how you're different from other addicts. You're looking for loopholes when you think that you're doing your recovery for somebody else instead of for yourself.

Nothing changes, if nothing changes. This is the wisdom of AA. If you don't change your life, if you don't learn new coping skills, if you don't ask for help, what will have changed? Why will this time be any different? "If you do what you've always done, you'll get what you've always gotten."[91] Ask yourself: will more lying, more isolating, and more of the same help you recover?

You can change your life. You can recover from addiction. You will do it by creating a new life where it's easier to not use.

The Importance of Self-Care

Self-care means making time to escape, relax, and reward yourself in ways that contribute to your long-term happiness. Taking better care of yourself is the essence of recovery. Take better care of yourself by making relaxation part of your life, by getting a good night's sleep, by eating right, and by having fun every once in a while. Recovery isn't about one big change. It's about lots of little changes.

A Story of Commitment

Wayne is a self-made millionaire who started a company that became a multinational corporation. Along the way, he developed a
crack addiction. Fortunately, he had the good sense to stop using
before he lost everything, and he went into treatment.

Wayne stayed in rehab for three months. When he came out, he
had the humility to go into a recovery home for six months. There he
shared a room with another recovering addict and was responsible
for the daily chores of the house. He had to cook, clean, do laundry,
you name it. That's commitment.

But the part of the story that really caught my attention was
this tiny detail. After he had been in recovery for a while, Wayne decided to go to a sporting event downtown. Before going, he planned
every step of what he would do once he left the event. He visualized
walking out of the exit, turning right, walking a block, turning right
again, and walking back to his recovery house.

Wayne planned his every move because he didn't want to leave
the event and find himself standing on the corner, wondering whether he should turn right or left. Without a plan, he could have ended
up taking the wrong direction, and find himself in the wrong part
of town. That's commitment.

Key Points

- You must change your life. You must create a new life where it's easier to not use. Otherwise all the factors that brought you to your addiction will eventually catch up with you again.
- Be completely honest. When you are honest, you don't give your addiction room to hide.
- Ask for help. Reach out and break the cycle of shame and isolation that perpetuates addiction.
- Relax every day. Tension is the most common cause of relapse.
- Don't make your own rules. Don't look for loopholes in recovery.

28

RELAPSE PREVENTION

The goal of recovery is not just to stop using drugs and alcohol, but to avoid relapsing in the future. In this chapter, I will explain the process of relapse and how to create a relapse prevention plan. But first, a story about relapse prevention. It's called "A Story of Recovery in Five Short Chapters." [92]

Chapter 1

I walk down a path. There is a deep hole, and I fall in by mistake. It takes me a long time to get out.

Chapter 2

I walk down a path. There is a deep hole. It's the same hole, but I fall in again.

Chapter 3

I walk down the same path. I see the hole, but again I fall in. This time I know where I am, and I get out quickly.

Chapter 4

I walk down the same path. The hole is there. But I walk around it.

Chapter 5

I take a different path where there is no hole.

The Process of Relapse

Relapse is a process, not an event. Relapse begins weeks or even months before the event of physical relapse. If you understand the process, you can catch yourself quickly before you go too far. There are three stages to relapse:[93]

- Emotional relapse
- Mental relapse
- Physical relapse

Emotional Relapse

In emotional relapse, you're not thinking about using. In fact, using is the furthest thing from your mind. But your emotions and behaviors are setting you up for a possible relapse in the future. The signs of emotional relapse are the following:

- Anxiety
- Intolerance
- Anger
- Defensiveness
- Mood swings
- Isolation
- Not asking for help
- Not going to meetings
- Poor eating habits
- Poor sleep habits

Because you're not consciously thinking about using at this stage, denial is a big part of emotional relapse. When someone suggests that you are setting yourself up for relapse, you become defensive.

Early Relapse Prevention

Early prevention involves recognizing the early warning signs. In the later stages of relapse, the pull of addiction gets stronger and the sequence of events moves faster and faster.

The basis of early relapse prevention is self-care. Identify that you're anxious, and practice mind-body relaxation. Recognize that you're isolating yourself, and ask for help. Acknowledge that your sleep habits are slipping, and take better care of yourself.

This is how relapse prevention fits into the five rules of recovery. You must change your life, and one of the things you must change is taking better care of yourself. Addicts are notoriously poor at self-care.

How do you shift from emotional to mental relapse? If you live too long in emotional relapse and don't take care of yourself, you will become emotionally exhausted. When you are exhausted, you will think of turning to your addiction to escape. When you begin to think about using, you will shift from emotional to mental relapse. In other words, your own actions during emotional relapse set you up for mental relapse.

Mental Relapse

During mental relapse, there's a war going on in your mind. Part of you wants to use, but part of you doesn't. In the early phase of mental relapse, you're idly thinking about using. But in the later phase, you're *definitely* thinking about using. The signs of mental relapse are the following:

- Thinking about people who you used with
- Fantasizing about using
- Hanging out with using friends
- Glamorizing past use
- Lying
- Planning a relapse around other people's schedules

Techniques for Dealing with Mental Urges

It gets harder to make the right choices as the pull of addiction gets stronger. But even in mental relapse there are a number of things you can do to stop the process.

Play the tape through. When you think about using, the fantasy is that you'll be able to control your use. This time, you'll just have one drink or one hit of cocaine. But play the tape through. One drink usually leads to two, which leads to more. You'll wake up the next day feeling disappointed in yourself. You may not be able to stop the next day. Your relationships will begin to suffer. You'll get caught in the same vicious cycle. When you play the tape through to its logical conclusion, using doesn't seem so appealing.

A common thought during mental relapse is that you can get away with using this time because no one will know. Perhaps your spouse is away for the weekend, or you're away on a trip. That's when your addiction will try to convince you that you don't have a big problem, and that you're doing your recovery just to please someone else.

Play the tape through. Remind yourself of the negative consequences you've already suffered, and the potential consequences that lie ahead if you relapse again. If you were able to control your use, you would have done it by now.

Play the positive tape through. Remind yourself of how much better you feel now that you've stopped using. Think of how nice it is that you don't have to lie. Your mind is clearer. You have more energy. Your mood is improving. Do you really want to blow all that?

Tell someone that you're having urges. Call someone in recovery and share what you're going through. The magic of sharing is that the minute you start to talk about what you're feeling, your urges begin to fade. They don't seem quite as big, and you don't feel as alone.

Distract yourself. When you think about using, do something to occupy yourself. Go to a meeting. Get up and go for a walk. Have a relaxation session. If you just sit there with your urges, you will give your mental relapse room to grow.

Give yourself 30 minutes. Most urges usually last less than 15 to 30 minutes. When you have an urge, it feels like eternity. But if you keep yourself busy and do something positive, it will pass. Once you've dealt with a few urges, you'll begin to feel confident that they won't last forever and that you can overcome them.

Do your recovery one day at a time. Be in the moment. Don't think about whether you can stay abstinent forever. That's a paralyzing thought. It's overwhelming even for people who've been in recovery a long time. If you're in the moment, you won't sabotage your recovery by thinking too far ahead.

One day at a time means matching your goals with your emotional strength. When you feel strong and motivated, tell yourself that you won't use for the next week or the next month. But when you're struggling – and those times will happen – tell yourself that you won't use for today, or for the next 30 minutes. Do your recovery in bite-sized chunks. Addiction is cunning and powerful, and you can't beat it all at once.

Jason is an alcoholic, who finds himself in rehab for the third time. His employer has made him sign a "last chance" agreement. If he messes up one more time, Jason will be fired. He only has one more chance at home too, and he knows it. There is a lot a stake, so he needs to figure out why he keeps relapsing. This is the story of how he got here.

After completing rehab the second time, Jason went to AA meetings three times a week. For the first five months, he did well. He didn't drink, and he had few urges to drink. That's not unusual. People are so relieved after they stop using that they don't struggle with their addiction. Jason went to AA meetings and told everyone how wonderful he felt. Rehab and AA had saved his life.

But then little problems started to creep in. He faced a few challenges that he could have overcome if he did the right thing. But he didn't. The first mistake he made was not telling his recovery group that he was struggling. He had been telling everyone that he was doing well, and now he was reluctant to tell them that he was having cravings. He told himself he didn't want to disappoint the others in the group or alarm his wife.

Jason broke the second rule of recovery. He wasn't being honest. His little white lies started eating him up. He could have prevented a relapse, had he only asked for help. But he broke the third rule of recovery.

Jason started to withdraw. He felt so uncomfortable about his lies that he started to go to fewer meetings. He was caught in a cycle of shame and isolation. He justified why he didn't need to go to meetings, and soon he was thinking about using. With this, he moved from emotional relapse to mental relapse. Jason broke the fifth rule of recovery. He was following his own advice, and making up his own rules.

With each passing day, the voice of his addiction grew stronger, until eventually, Jason reached the point where he did what was familiar and wrong instead of what was new and right. Within a month of starting to struggle, he had relapsed. That's why he ended up with a "last chance" agreement and a strained marriage.

Fortunately Jason learned a lesson from his relapse. He went through rehab, went to AA, and learned to ask for help. He practiced being completely honest, and turned his life around.

You Can't Eliminate Thoughts of Using

No matter how well you do in recovery, you will still have occasional thoughts of using. There are two kinds of using thoughts. There are "normal thoughts," which are brief and easy to let go. They don't necessarily mean you're going to relapse.

The other kind are dangerous thoughts of using, which are different. They are difficult to dismiss. They become stronger over time, and they often involve glamorizing past use. If you have these thoughts, stop whatever you're doing and ask for help. Be completely honest. Increase your relaxation sessions, and practice self-care. Relapse is not inevitable.

The distinguishing features of normal using thoughts are that they are brief, easy to let go, and occur infrequently. They don't have the same pull as mental relapse.

Once you have given your lower brain a taste of addiction, it will never forget it. This explains why you have occasional thoughts of using, even though you're horrified at the idea of relapse. The answer goes back to the two parts of the brain. Normal using thoughts come from the primitive brain, which is devoted to pleasure and survival. Once it has tasted the buzz of addiction, it will never forget it. Over time, your memories will fade. But they will never go away completely.

The Final Step: Physical Relapse

Once you start thinking about using, you can move from mental relapse to physical relapse in the blink of an eye. You drive to the liquor store, or meet your dealer, and your fate is sealed. It's hard to stop the process of relapse at this point. This is not where you should focus your efforts in relapse prevention.

If you recognize the early warning signs, and practice self-care, you can prevent physical relapses from happening. Don't reduce your relapse prevention to the simple act of not using. There is an enormous difference between abstinence and recovery. Create a new life where you will not be triggered, and life will be a lot easier.

Dealing with Social Events

Social events are common sources of trouble in early recovery. Many relapse prevention strategies don't work if you're already at a social event. Once you are there, and if you can't avoid the event, then you need different strategies.

Immediately get a drink in your hand. The first thing you should do when you go to a social event is get a non-alcoholic drink in your hand. It is a prop that gives you something to hold onto, and makes you feel like you belong. If you walk around with nothing in your hand, people will ask if they can get you a drink, which will put you in an awkward situation.

Be the first to order a drink when you're in a group. Suppose you're at a work function, and the waiter comes by to order drinks. Be the first to put your order in. If you wait until everyone else has ordered, you may feel peer pressure to order what they are having.

Never leave your drink unattended. Never leave a drink and assume that it will be safe when you return. Someone may have thought they were doing you a favor and freshened it up with alcohol.

Leave parties early. All the heavy drinking usually happens at the end of a party. The main reason people hang around at the end is to drink heavily. Therefore make sure you leave before that crowd gets started. If your recovery is solid, you might not be triggered by moderate drinking. But you will probably be triggered by heavy drinking.

Always have an exit strategy. Sometimes, even moderate drinking can make you feel uncomfortable. If that happens, leave an event quickly. Don't pretend that you're all right. Thank your host and leave.

If you're at the event with a friend, make sure they agreed to your exit strategy beforehand, or that you don't rely on them for transportation. Don't put yourself in a position where you have to hang around when you feel uncomfortable and triggered.

Try not to have social events at your place in the beginning, because you'll have no exit strategy. You'll be at the mercy of everyone else's schedule, waiting for your guests to leave before you can have your space back.

Avoidance is always an option. In the early stages of recovery, the best relapse prevention strategy is avoidance. You don't have to go to social events if you feel uncomfortable. This is especially true for the first year. Later, as you develop better coping skills, you will want to re-engage in the world.

But there will still be times when you will feel vulnerable, when the mix of people is too much to handle, or when your emotional reserves are low. At those times, remember that avoidance is still an option. Sometimes the best form of self-care is avoidance.

There are three kinds of people at social events. The vast majority of people don't care what you're drinking. As long as you've got a drink in your hand, they're happy.

A smaller group of people will be a little curious about why you're not drinking alcohol. They won't want to know your life story.

They just want to know why you're not drinking today. Any explanation will be good enough for them. You can say you're driving, you're tired, you want to lose weight, or you just don't feel like a drink.

This leaves the smallest group of people, those who push drinks. They are the ones who insist that you join them in a drink. And they are almost always problem drinkers. Therefore, put what they say in perspective. One of the reasons problem drinkers push drinks is because they feel uncomfortable when other people drink less than they do.

If you follow these simple strategies, you can get back to socializing without too much discomfort. With a little practice, you'll be able to enjoy yourself even more than you did before.

Key Points

- There are three stages to relapse: emotional, mental, and physical.
- In emotional relapse, you're not thinking about using. But your emotions and behaviors are setting you up for a possible relapse in the future.
- If you stay in emotional relapse too long, you will become uncomfortable or exhausted, and you will think of using to escape.
- There is an enormous difference between abstinence and recovery. Focus your efforts on early relapse prevention instead of on trying to avoid physical relapse.
- The key to relapse prevention is good self-care.

29

SURVIVE POST-ACUTE WITHDRAWAL

There are two stages to withdrawal. The first stage, acute withdrawal, occurs once you stop using drugs or alcohol, and can last up to a few weeks. The second stage, post-acute withdrawal syndrome (PAWS), is more important because it can last up to two years.

Post-acute withdrawal is a common cause of relapse. If you expect that you will fully recover after just a few weeks of quitting drugs and alcohol, you'll be caught off guard. But with a few survival strategies you can get through this. In this chapter you will learn the symptoms of post-acute withdrawal and how to get through it.

What Causes Withdrawal?

Your brain works like a spring. The spring represents the neurotransmitters in your brain. When you use drugs and alcohol, this pushes down the spring and depresses the production of certain neurotransmitters. When you stop using, you take the weight off the spring, and the spring bounces back producing a surge of neurotransmitters and the symptoms of withdrawal.

During the acute stage of withdrawal, some drugs produce significant symptoms, for example alcohol and heroin, while other drugs such as marijuana and cocaine produce very few. The symptoms of acute withdrawal tend to be mostly physical, and include tremors, sweating, and nausea. In severe cases, acute withdrawal can also lead to seizures and heart attacks. (For more information on acute withdrawal and its potential dangers refer to the supplementary website www.AddictionsAndRecovery.org.)

After initial withdrawal, the spring then begins to bounce up and down as it gradually goes back to equilibrium. During this time, your neurotransmitters are out of balance, which produces the symptoms of post-acute withdrawal. Once your brain chemistry returns to equilibrium, the symptoms will fade away.

In acute withdrawal every drug and person is different. Whereas during post-acute withdrawal, the situation is reversed. Most people experience similar post-acute withdrawal symptoms regardless of what drug they used. The symptoms tend to be less physical and more emotional and psychological. Also the danger of withdrawal disappears after the first few weeks.

Post-acute withdrawal usually lasts for two years. This is one of the most important things you need to remember about post-acute withdrawal. If you're up for the challenge, you can get through this. But if you think that post-acute withdrawal will only last for a few months, you'll get caught off guard. And when you are disappointed, you are more likely to relapse.

The Symptoms of Post-Acute Withdrawal

The most common symptoms of post-acute withdrawal are the following:
- Mood swings
- Anxiety
- Irritability
- Tiredness
- Variable energy
- Low enthusiasm
- Variable concentration
- Disturbed sleep

Post-acute withdrawal feels like a rollercoaster. In the beginning, your symptoms will change minute to minute, and hour to hour. Later, your symptoms will disappear for a few weeks or months, only to return again. With time, the good stretches will grow longer, but the bad periods can be just as intense and last just as long.

Each episode of post-acute withdrawal usually lasts for a few days. There is no obvious trigger for most episodes. Some days, you will wake up feeling irritable and exhausted for no good reason. If you take care of yourself, the symptoms will lift after a few days just as quickly as they started. Gradually, you'll become confident that you can get through post-acute withdrawal because you'll understand that each episode is limited.

What's the difference between post-acute withdrawal and a bad day? The symptoms are similar. But a bad day usually happens for a reason, whereas post-acute withdrawal can occur for no reason at all.

Post-acute withdrawal days follow a predictable pattern. They are more frequent in the early days of recovery and less frequent later on. Bad days, on the other hand, happen with roughly the same frequency, regardless of what stage of recovery you're in.

How to Survive Post-Acute Withdrawal

Two years can feel like a long time if you're in a rush. You can't hurry recovery. But you can get through it one day at a time.

Be patient. If you try to rush post-acute withdrawal, or resent it, you'll become exhausted. When you're exhausted, you will think of turning to your addiction to escape. Post-acute withdrawal symptoms are a sign that your brain is recovering. Don't resent them. Even after one year, you are still only halfway there.

Go with the flow. Withdrawal symptoms are uncomfortable. But the more you resent them, the worse they feel. You will have lots of good days over the next two years. Enjoy them. You will also have a few bad days. On those days, don't try to do too much. Take care of yourself, focus on your recovery, and you'll come out the other end.

Here is a common scenario. One day you'll wake up, and the minute your feet hit the floor you'll know this is going to be a bad day. You'll have slept badly. You'll be in a bad mood, and your energy will be low.

The wrong way to deal with these symptoms is to plow through your day and ignore how you feel. Doing this will use up the little physical reserve that you have, and you'll become exhausted.

The right way to deal with post-acute withdrawal is to understand that this is a down day, and lower your expectations. Go to a meeting, share how you're feeling, relax, get a good night's sleep, and know that in a day or two you'll start to feel better again.

Practice self-care. Give yourself lots of little breaks over the next two years. Tell yourself, "What I am doing is enough." Be good to yourself. This is what most addicts can't do, and what you must learn in recovery. Recovery is the opposite of addiction. At times, you'll have little enthusiasm for anything. Understand this, and don't overbook your life. Give yourself permission to focus on your recovery.

Remember that every relapse, no matter how small, undoes the gains your brain has made during recovery. Without abstinence, everything will fall apart. With abstinence, everything is possible.

Key Points

- Post-acute withdrawal symptoms include mood swings, variable energy, and variable concentration.
- Your symptoms will gradually improve over two years.
- Measure your progress on a monthly basis instead of weekly so that you don't get frustrated.
- Take care of yourself, relax every day, and you will get through this.

30

FINAL THOUGHTS

"You must be the change you wish to see in the world." [94]
– MAHATMA MOHANDAS GANDHI

I would like to leave you with a few final thoughts about the role of mind-body relaxation in happiness. In more than twenty years of practicing medicine I have learned that tension is the universal denominator in most people's problems. I've tried to summarize this fact in what I call my "four laws of happiness."

1. **Knowledge is not enough for happiness.** Intelligent people who are successful in many areas of life are often unhappy. The standard approach to self-help is to give people more information hoping this will lead to change. But that's usually the easy part. Most people already know what they're doing wrong. The hard part of being happy and improving your life is not repeating the same mistakes.

2. **Tension is the biggest preventable cause of unhappiness.** Tension affects every aspect of life. It damages everything from your self-esteem to your relationships. It leads to negative thinking and contributes to anxiety, depression, and addiction. It directly or indirectly contributes to most diseases. Few factors have a greater impact on life than tension.

3. **Tension is the main obstacle to change.** Tension not only makes you unhappy, it keeps you stuck in unhappiness. When you're tense, you tend to do what's familiar and wrong instead of what's new and right. This is why knowledge alone is not enough. When

you're tense, it's hard to let go of your ego and fears to make room for change.

4. Reducing tension is key to improving your life. Mind-body relaxation is the foundation on which all other coping skills are built. Think of it this way. There are many coping skills you need to be happy. If you learn them all but don't learn how to relax, you still won't do well, because when you're tense you will continue to repeat what's familiar and wrong.

On the other hand, if you learn only one new coping skill – how to relax – you'll still be happier, because everything is easier when you're relaxed. If there is anything else you must learn in order to be happy, you'll see it more clearly and deal with it more effectively when you're more relaxed.

Considering that relaxation is so important, it's interesting that it's so rarely taught. The further we go in school the more specialized information we learn. But the really important stuff, like what will make us happy, is hardly ever taught. Why is that?

The importance of mind-body relaxation has only recently been recognized in medicine. As recently as 1950, Hans Selye, pioneering researcher on the physiology of stress, had to coin the words *le stress* and *der stress*. Incredibly, many languages didn't have a word for stress at the time. He also coined the word *stressor*, which has become part of our vocabulary.

In Herbert Benson's popular book, *The Relaxation Response*, he wrote, "Western science had not, in the nineteen sixties, begun to entertain the possibility that physical problems might be rooted in mental or emotional activity, or that stress as a phenomenon could engender demonstrable physical problems."[95]

It's hard to believe, but just a few years ago, doctors dismissed the connection between the body and mind. They didn't believe that your emotional state could cause physical problems, or that physical problems could hurt your emotional state. The few doctors who dared challenge that dogma did so at considerable risk to their professional careers.

Medicine has come so far in such a short period of time that it is hard to imagine how confidently ignorant we once were. Yet for thousands of years ordinary people have known that they could improve their health and happiness by relaxing their body and mind.

I believe that mind-body relaxation will play an even bigger role in the future of medicine. Good medicine is not just about treating illness; but about healing people. And healing involves helping the body help itself. It involves overcoming the scourge of tension and treating the mind, body, and soul as one.

RESOURCES

Books

- *The Anxiety and Phobia Workbook, 4th ed.* Edmund J Bourne. New Harbinger Publications, 2005.
- Better Brains. *Scientific American.* Sept 2003.
- *Cognitive Therapy and the Emotional Disorders.* Aaron T. Beck. Penguin Press, 1979.
- *Eight Weeks to Optimum Health: A Proven Program for Taking Full Advantage of Your Body's Natural Healing Power.* Andrew Weil. Ballantine Books, 1998.
- *Feeling Good.* David D. Burns. William Morrow, 1980.
- *Full Catastrophe Living.* Jon Kabat-Zin. Delta, 1990.
- *Mindfulness in Plain English.* Henepola Gunartana. Wisdom, 1991.
- *Mind Over Mood.* Dennis Greenberger and Christine A Padesky. The Guilford Press, 1995.
- *Perfect Health: The Complete Mind/Body Guide.* Deepak Chopra. Harmony, 1991.
- *The Physical and Psychological Effects of Meditation.* Michael Murphy and Steven Donovan. Institute of Noetic Sciences, 1999.
- *The Relaxation Response.* Herbert Benson and Miriam Klipper. Avon, 2000.
- *The Seven Principles for Making Marriage Work.* John M. Gottman and Nan Silver. Three Rivers Press, 1999.
- *The Six Pillars of Self-Esteem.* Nathaniel Branden. Bantam, 1994.
- *The Way of Zen.* Alan Watts. Vintage, 1989.

Websites and Organizations

American Institute of Stress
A not-for-profit organization established in 1978 as a clearinghouse for stress-related information. Its founding members included Hans Selye, Linus Pauling, Alvin Toffler, Bob Hope, Michael DeBakey, and Herbert Benson.
www.stress.org

The Beck Institute for Cognitive Therapy
Founded by Dr. Aaron Beck, the father of modern cognitive therapy, and his daughter, Dr. Judith Beck.
www.beckinstitute.org

The Chopra Center
A health and wellness program that uses mind-body relaxation and meditation among other things.
www.chopra.com

The Mind/Body Medical Institute
Founded by Dr. Herbert Benson, author of *The Relaxation Response.*
www.mbmi.org

Mindfulness in Medicine, Health Care, and Society
Founded by Dr. Jon Kabat-Zin, whose meditation program is used in a number of health care programs.
www.umassmed.edu/cfm

National Association of Cognitive Behavioral Therapists
A database of all certified cognitive behavioral therapists.
www.nacbt.org

National Center for Complementary and Alternative Medicine
Information on alternative medicine from a member of the National Institutes of Health.
nccam.nih.gov

National Center for PTSD
Part of US Department of Veterans Affairs
www.ncptsd.va.gov

National Institutes of Mental Health
Information and programs on the entire range of mental health issues.
www.nimh.nih.gov

Preventive Medicine Institute
The Preventive Medicine Research Institute offers a medically corroborated program for treating heart disease that uses exercise, nutrition, and mind-body relaxation.
www.pmri.org

Dr. Andrew Weil
A health and wellness program that uses mind-body relaxation among other things.
www.drweil.com

ABOUT THE AUTHOR

Dr. Melemis is a leading expert in addictions and mood disorders. He was born in Toronto, has a PhD and MD from the University of Toronto, and has a post-doctoral fellowship from the University of California at Berkeley. He has received the honor of Fellow of the Royal Society of Medicine. Dr. Melemis has lectured widely to the public and to health professionals, and has been interviewed for television, radio, and print.

ACKNOWLEDGMENTS

I'd like to thank my patients, who have taught me so much. My dear friends, Bethann Colle and Michael Clark read the manuscript many times and provided invaluable suggestions. Thank you to my assistant, Crystal Winegarden, who is amazing. Special thanks to my wife Cindy for making it all fun.

It has been a pleasure to have worked with a number of people on this book. The editorial consultant was Ann Dowsett Johnston. Copy editing and indexing was by Wendy Thomas. Book design was by Jennifer Stimson. The author's photo is by Edward Gajdel.

Finally, it's an honor to thank my parents Georgia and Anthony for their love and support over the years. Thank you to everyone.

REFERENCES

1   The Dalai Lama and Howard C. Cutler, *The Art of Happiness* (Riverhead Books, 1998), pp. 13, 15.

2   Attributed to Danzae Pace.

3   The Dalai Lama, *How to Practice: The Way to a Meaningful Life.* Translated and edited by Jeffrey Hopkins. (Pocket Books, 2002), p. 97.

4   Santideva, *The Way of the Bodhisattva: A Translation of the Bodhicharyavatara* (Chapter 5) (Shambhala, 1997).

5   Epictetus, *The Enchiridion* (trans. The Handbook).

6   Some of this material is based on the works of A.T. Beck, A.J. Rush, B.F. Shaw, and G. Emery, *Cognitive Therapy of Depression* (Guilford Press, 1979) and David Burns, *Feeling Good* (Quill, 2000).

7   A.T. Beck, A.J. Rush, B.F. Shaw, and G. Emery, *Cognitive Therapy of Depression* (Guilford Press, 1979), p. 11.

8   Mark Twain, *Pudd'nhead Wilson's New Calendar.* Mark Twain Quotations, http://www.twainquotes.com/Wrinkles.html.

9   Karen Armstrong, *Buddha* (Viking, 2001), p. 112.

10 Lao-Tzu, *Tao-te-ching.* Bk. 1, Chapter 67.

11 MD Lieberman, NI Eisenberger, MJ Crockett, SM Tom, JH Pfeifer, and BM Way, "Putting feelings into words: affect labeling disrupts amygdala activity in response to affective stimuli," *Psychol Sci* 2007 May;18(5):421–28.

12 Watts, *The Way of Zen*, p. 93.

13 Lawrence LeShan, *How to Meditate* (Little Brown, 1974), p. 55.

14 S.W. Lazar, G. Bush, R.L. Gollub, G.L. Fricchione, G. Khalsa, and H. Benson, "Functional brain mapping of the relaxation response and meditation," *Neuroreport* 2000 May 15;11(7):1581–85.

15 R.J. Davidson, J. Kabat-Zinn, J. Schumacher, M. Rosenkranz, D. Muller, S.F. Santorelli, F. Urbanowski, A. Harrington, K. Bonus, and J.F. Sheridan, "Alterations in brain and immune

function produced by mindfulness meditation," *Psychosomatic medicine* 2003 Jul-Aug;65(4):564–70.

16 Dhammapada, *The Sayings of the Buddha*. Translated by Thomas Byron (Shambhala, 1993).

17 Lao Tzu, *Tao-te-ching*.

18 Fukanzazengi. In Teachings of the Buddha. ed. Jack Kornfield (Shambhala, 1996).

19 Voltaire, *Philosophical Dictionary*, "Dramatic Art." 1764.

20 Michelle Conlin, "Meditation," *BusinessWeek* Aug. 23, 2004. Lisa Cullen, "How to Get Smarter One Breath at a Time," *Time* Jan. 16, 2006. "A post-modern proctoid," *The Economist* April 15, 2006.

21 Attributed to William James.

22 Aaron T. Beck, *Cognitive Therapy and the Emotional Disorders* (Penguin Press, 1979).

23 David Burns, *Feeling Good* (Quill, 2000).

24 The Oracle of Delphi was counsel to the ancient world for more than a thousand years. These words were written over its entrance.

25 Carlos Castaneda, *Journey to Ixtlan* (Simon and Schuster, 1972), p. 184.

26 Fukanzazengi. In *Teachings of the Buddha*. ed. Jack Kornfield (Shambhala, 1996).

27 Andy Warhol (1928–87), U.S. pop artist. Exhibition catalogue, Oct.-Nov. 1966, ICA, Boston.

28 Nathaniel Branden, *The Six Pillars of Self-Esteem* (Bantam, 1994).

29 Alan Watts, *The Way of Zen*, p. 10.

30 Albert Schweitzer. Quoted in Norman Cousins, *Anatomy of an Illness as Perceived by the Patient* (Bantam, 1991), p. 69.

31 E.S. Epel, EH Blackburn, J. Lin, FS Dhabhar, N.E. Adler, J.D. Morrow, and R.M. Cawthon, "Accelerated telomere shortening in response to life stress," *Proc Natl Acad Sci U S A* 2004 Dec 7;101(49):17312–15.

32 Michael Murphy and Steven Donovan, *The Physical and Psychological Effects of Meditation: A Review of Contemporary Research with a Comprehensive Bibliography 1931–1996.* (Institute of Noetic Sciences, 1999).

33 Norman Cousins, *Head First: The Biology of Hope* (Dutton, 1989), p. 96.

34 C. Patel, M.G. Marmot, D.J. Terry, M. Carruthers, B. Hunt, and M. Patel, "Trial of relaxation in reducing coronary risk: four year follow up," *Br Med J (Clin Res Ed)* 1985 Apr 13; 290(6475):1103–6.

35 A. Castillo-Richmond, R.H. Schneider, C.N. Alexander, R. Cook, H. Myers, S. Nidich, C. Haney, M. Rainforth, and J. Salerno, "Effects of stress reduction on carotid atherosclerosis in hypertensive African Americans," *Stroke* 2000 Mar; 31(3):568–73.

36 R.J. Davidson, J. Kabat-Zinn, J. Schumacher, M. Rosenkranz, D. Muller, S.F. Santorelli, F. Urbanowski, A Harrington, K Bonus, and JF Sheridan, "Alterations in brain and immune function produced by mindfulness meditation," *Psychosomatic medicine* 2003 Jul–Aug; 65(4):564–70.

37 R.H. Schneider, C.N Alexander, F. Staggers, M. Rainforth, J.W. Salerno, A. Hartz, S. Arndt, V.A. Barnes, and S.I. Nidich, "Long-term effects of stress reduction on mortality in persons >/=55 years of age with systemic hypertension," *Am J Cardiol* 2005 May 1;95(9):1060–64.

38 G.S. Berns, J. Chappelow, M. Cekic, et al., "Neurobiological substrates of dread," *Science* 5 May 2006: Vol. 312. no. 5774, p. 754–58.

39 J.L. Harte, G.H. Eifert, and R. Smith, "The effects of running and meditation on beta-endorphin, corticotropin-releasing hormone and cortisol in plasma, and on mood," *Biol Psychol* 1995 Jun; 40(3):251–65.

40 J. Kabat-Zinn, L. Lipworth, and R. Burney, "The clinical use of mindfulness meditation for the self-regulation of chronic pain," *J Behav Med* 1985 Jun; 8(2):163–90.

41 W.E. Mehling, K.A. Hamel, M. Acree, N. Byl, and F.M. Hecht, "Randomized, controlled trial of breath therapy for patients with chronic low-back pain," *Altern Ther Health Med* 2005 Jul–Aug; 11(4):44–52.

42 K.H. Kaplan, D.L. Goldenberg, and M. Galvin-Nadeau, "The impact of a meditation-based stress reduction program on fibromyalgia," *Gen Hosp Psychiatry* 1993 Sep; 15(5):284–89.

43 J.A. Astin, S.L. Shapiro, D.M. Eisenberg, and K.L. Forys, "Mind-body medicine: state of the science, implications for practice," *J Am Board Fam Pract* 2003 Mar-Apr; 16(2):131–47.

44 R.D. Vorona, M.P. Winn, T.W. Babineau, B.P. Eng, H.R. Feldman, and J.C. Ware, "Overweight and obese patients in a primary care population report less sleep than patients with a normal body mass index," *Arch Intern Med* 2005 Jan 10;165(1):25–30.

45 Traditional proverb.

46 John M. Gottman and Nan Silver, *The Seven Principles for Making Marriage Work* (Three Rivers Press, 1999). John M. Gottman and Joan DeClaire, *The Relationship Cure* (Three Rivers Press, 2001).

47 Gottman and Silver, *The Seven Principles for Making Marriage Work*, p. 27.

48 Gottman and Silver, *The Seven Principles for Making Marriage Work*, p. 40.

49 The Dalai Lama, *How to Practice: The Way to a Meaningful Life*. Translated and edited by Jeffrey Hopkins. (Pocket Books, 2002), p. 70.

50 Dalai Lama, referred to in Jon Kabat-Zinn, Wherever You Go, There You Are (Hyperion, 1994), p. 168.

51 Buddhist wisdom.

52 J.H. Fowler, N.A. Christakis, "Dynamic spread of happiness in a large social network: longitudinal analysis over 20 years in the Framingham Heart Study," *British Medical Journal*, 2008 Dec 4;337:a2338.

53 Alan W. Watts, *The Way of Zen* (Vintage, 1957), p. 199.

54 National Comorbidity Survey Lifetime Prevalence Estimates, http://www.hcp.med.harvard.edu/ncs/.

55 A. Joseph Campbell, *Reflections on the Art of Loving: A Joseph Campbell Companion*, ed. Diane K. Osbon (Harper Perennial, 1991), p. 52.

56 J. Kabat-Zinn, A.O. Massion, J. Kristeller, L.G. Peterson, K.E. Fletcher, L. Pbert, W.R. Lenderking, and S.F. Santorelli, "Effectiveness of a meditation-based stress reduction program in the treatment of anxiety disorders," *Am J Psychiatry* 1992 Jul;149(7):936–43.

57 Henry David Thoreau, *Walden Pond*. "Where I Lived, and What I Lived For," 1854.

58 N. Breslau, R.C. Kessler, H.D. Chilcoat, L.R. Schultz, GC Davis, and P Andreski, "Trauma and posttraumatic stress disorder in the community: The 1996 Detroit Area Survey of Trauma," *Archives of General Psychiatry* 55 (1998): 626–32.

59 B.P. Dohrenwend, J.B. Turner, N.A. Turse, B.G. Adams, K.C. Koen, and R. Marshall, "The psychological risk of Vietnam for U.S. veterans: A revisit with new data and methods," *Science.* 2006; 313(5789):979–82.

60 J. Sareen, S.L. Belik, T.O. Afifi, G.J. Asmundson, B.J. Cox, and M.B. Stein, "Canadian military personnel's population attributable fractions of mental disorders and mental health service use associated with combat and peacekeeping operations," *Am J Public Health.* 2008 Dec;98(12):2191-8. Epub 2008 Oct 15.

61 B. Manville, *Cool, Hip & Sober: 88 Ways to Beat Booze and Drugs* (A Forge Book, 2003), p. 228.

62 Elizabeth Wurtzel, Prozac Nation (Riverhead Trade, 2002), p. 294.

63 R.C. Kessler, K.A. McGonagle, S. Zhao, C.B. Nelson, M. Hughes, S. Eshleman, H.U. Wittchen, and K.S. Kendler, "Lifetime and 12-month prevalence of DSM-III-R psychiatric disorders in the United States. Results from the National Comorbidity Survey," *Arch Gen Psychiatry.* 1994 Jan;51(1):8–19.

64 R.C. Kessler, P. Berglund, O. Demler, R. Jin, D. Koretz, K.R. Merikangas, A.J. Rush, E.E. Walters, and P.S. Wang, "The epidemiology of major depressive disorder: results from the National Comorbidity Survey Replication (NCS-R)," *JAMA*. 2003 Jun 18;289(23):3095–105.

65 C.D. Mathers, D. Loncar, "Projections of global mortality and burden of disease from 2002 to 2030," *PLoS Med* 2006 November; 3 (11): e442.

66 These are the combined criteria of the American Psychiatric Association (DSM-IV) and the World Health Organization (ICD-10). The DSM requires that you have at least five of the above symptoms for at least two weeks before you meet the criteria for depression. The ICD requires that you have at least three symptoms to meet the criteria of mild depression but does not set a time limit. Some doctors feel that two weeks is too brief, and that many people feel sad for two weeks without being depressed.

67 B.J. Sadock, V.A. Sadock, *Kaplan & Sadock's Synopsis of Psychiatry 9th ed.* (Philadelphia: Lippincott Williams & Wilkins 2003), p. 552.

68 K.S. Kendler, M. Gatz, C.O. Gardner, and N.L. Pedersen, "A Swedish national twin study of lifetime major depression," *Am J Psychiatry* 2006 Jan;163(1):109–14.

69 K.S. Kendler, S.H. Aggen, "Time, memory and the heritability of major depression," *Psychological medicine* 2001, vol. 31, no5, pp. 923–28.

70 M.A. Schuckit, J.E. Tipp, M. Bergman, W. Reich, V.M. Hesselbrock, and T.L. Smith, "Comparison of induced and independent major depressive disorders in 2,945 alcoholics," *American Journal Psychiatry*. 1997 Jul;154(7):948–57.

71 G.B. Bovasso, "Cannabis abuse as a risk factor for depressive symptoms," *American Journal Psychiatry*. 2001 Dec;158(12):2033–37.

72 G.C. Patton, C. Coffey, J.B. Carlin, L. Degenhardt, M. Lynskey, and W. Hall, "Cannabis use and mental health in young

people: cohort study," *British Medical Journal.* 2002 Nov 23;325(7374):1195–98.

73 M.A. Schuckit, J.E. Tipp, M. Bergman, W. Reich, V.M. Hesselbrock, and T.L. Smith, "Comparison of induced and independent major depressive disorders in 2,945 alcoholics," *American Journal Psychiatry.* 1997 Jul;154(7):948–57.

74 R.C. Kessler, W.T. Chiu, O. Demler, and E.E. Walters, "Prevalence, severity, and comorbidity of twelve-month DSM-IV disorders in the National Comorbidity Survey Replication (NCS-R)," *Archives of General Psychiatry,* 2005 Jun;62(6):617–27.

75 A.T. Beck, A.J. Rush, B.F. Shaw, and G. Emery, *Cognitive Therapy of Depression* (Guilford Press, 1979), p. 124.

76 S.H. Ma and J.D. Teasdale, "Mindfulness-based cognitive therapy for depression: replication and exploration of differential relapse prevention effects," *J Consult Clin Psychol* 2004 Feb; 72(1):31–40.

77 B.A. Arnow and M.J. Constantino, "Effectiveness of psychotherapy and combination treatment for chronic depression," *J Clin Psychol.* 2003 Aug;59(8):893–905.

78 K. Linde, C.D. Mulrow, M. Berner, and M. Egger, "St John's wort for depression," *Cochrane Database Syst Rev.* 2005 Apr 18;(2):CD000448.

79 The American Institute of Stress, http://www.stress.org/job.htm.

80 Edward Albee, Zoo Story (Plume, 1997)

81 These are the combined criteria of the American Psychiatric Association (DSM-IV) and the World Health Organization (ICD-10).

82 C.A. Prescott and K.S. Kendler, "Genetic and environmental contributions to alcohol abuse and dependence in a population-based sample of male twins," *American Journal Psychiatry* 1999 Jan;156(1):34–40.

83 M.A. Enoch and D. Goldman, "The genetics of alcoholism and alcohol abuse," *Current Psychiatry Reports* 2001 Apr;3(2):144–51.

84 K.R. Merikangas, M. Stolar, D.E. Stevens, J. Goulet, M.A. Preisig, B. Fenton, H. Zhang, S.S. O'Malley, and B.J. Rounsaville, "Familial transmission of substance use disorders," *Archives General Psychiatry* 1998 Nov;55(11):973–79.

85 C.Y. Li, X. Mao, L. Wei, "Genes and common pathways underlying drug addiction," *PLoS Comput Biol.* 2008 Jan;4(1):e2. Epub 2007 Nov 20.

86 Napoleon Hill, The Law of Success in Sixteen Lessons (BNPublishing 2008), p 404.

87 H. Benson and R.K. Wallace, "Decreased Drug Abuse with Transcendental Meditation: A Study of 1862 Subjects," Congressional Record, 92nd Congress, 1st session, June 1971, Serial #92-1.

88 M. Shafil, R. Lavely, and R. Jaffe, "Meditation and the prevention of drug abuse," *American Journal of Psychiatry* 1975 (312): 942–45.

89 P. Gelderloos, K.G. Walton, D.W. Orme-Johnson, and C.N. Alexander, "Effectiveness of the Transcendental Meditation program in preventing and treating substance misuse: a review," *Int J Addict* 1991 Mar; 26(3):293–325.

90 A.N. Elias and A.F. Wilson, "Serum hormonal concentrations following transcendental meditation–potential role of gamma aminobutyric acid," *Med Hypotheses* 1995 Apr; 44(4):287–91.

91 AA wisdom.

92 Based on anonymous story from AA..

93 T. Gorski and M. Miller, *Counseling for Relapse Prevention* (Herald Publishing, 1982). T. Gorski and M. Miller, *Staying Sober: A Guide for Relapse Prevention* (Independence Press, 1986).

94 Attributed to Mohandas Gandhi.

95 Herbert Benson, *The Relaxation Response* (Whole Care, 2000), p. xiv.

INDEX

CONTACT INFORMATION

Visit the book website at
www.IWantToChangeMyLife.org

Supplementary material is available at
www.AnxietyDepressionHealth.org
www.AddictionsAndRecovery.org
www.CognitiveTherapyGuide.org
www.StressRelaxationGuide.org

Send your thoughts to
contact@IWantToChangeMyLife.org.

I Want To Change My Life is published by Modern Therapies.
www.ModernTherapies.com